Chiropractic Unleashed

The Ultimate Guide to Spinal Health

Mei Lin Zhang

Xspurts.com

A New Zealand Designed Product

Other Versions Available

Why limit yourself to just one format?

This book is now available in physical, digital, and audiobook options.

Choose the way you love to read and dive into the story today. You won't regret it!

Digital ISBN: 9781776968312
Physical ISBN: 9781776968305
Audio ISBN:

To obtain a different format of this book at a discounted price, please get in touch with us at:

http://isbn.xspurts.com/

Contents

Have Questions / Comments?

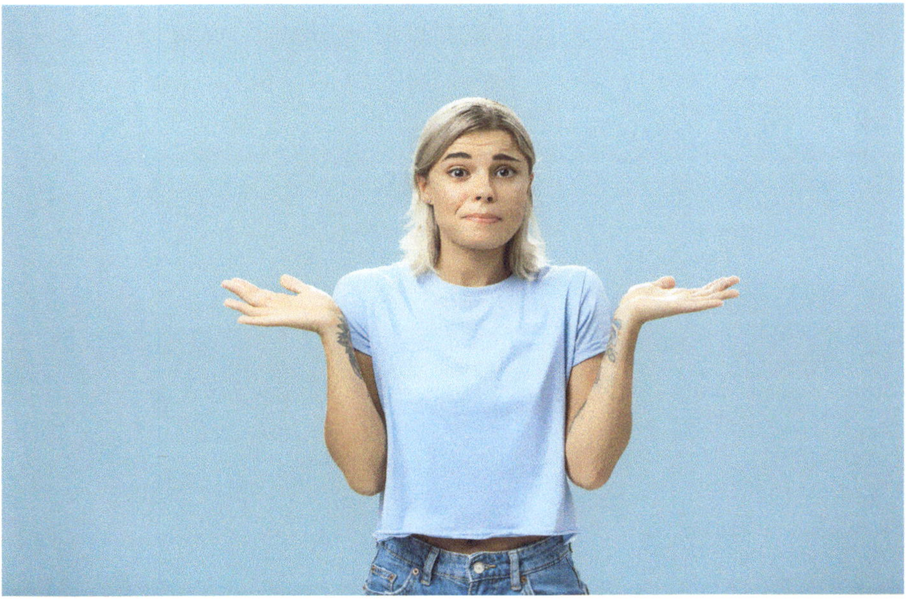

This book was designed to cover as much information as possible, but I know I have probably missed something, or some new amazing discovery has just come out.

If you notice something missing or have a question that I failed to answer, please get in touch and let me know. If I can, I will email you an answer and also update the book so others can also benefit from it.

Thanks For Being Awesome :)

Submit Your Questions / Comments At:

https://questions.xspurts.com

Get Free Stuff

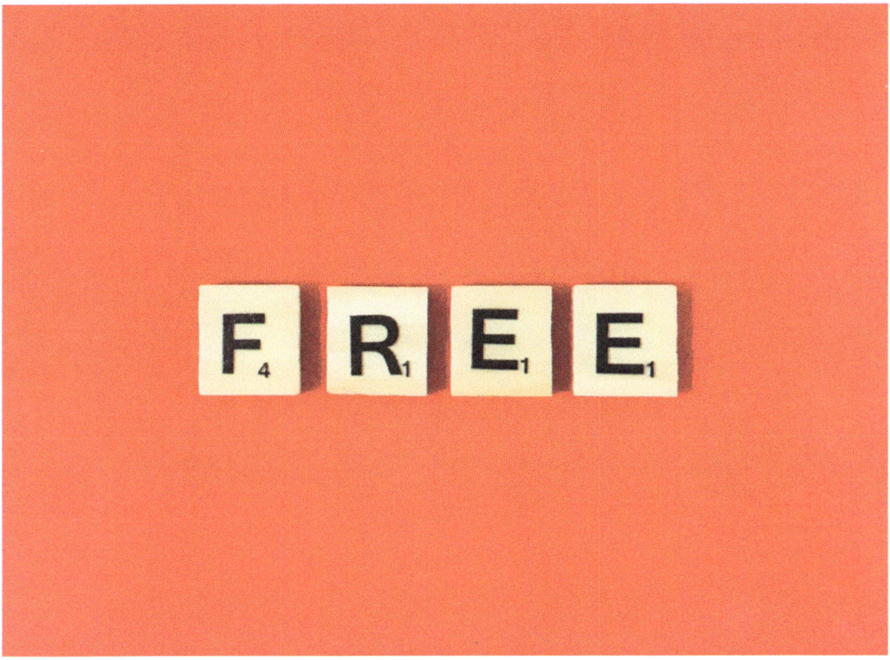

We love writing and have produced a huge number of books.

For being one of our amazing readers, we would love to offer you more books we have created, 100% free.

To claim this limited time special offer, simply go to the site below and enter your name and email address.

You will then receive loads (as we love our readers so much :) of our great books, content and audio direct to your email account, 100% free!

Get Loads of FREE Stuff at:

https://free.xspurts.com

Chapter One

Introduction to Chiropractic

Chiropractic is a form of complementary medicine that focuses on the diagnosis, treatment, and prevention of musculoskeletal disorders, particularly those that affect the spine. Chiropractors use a variety of manual techniques, including spinal manipulation and adjustment, to relieve pain and improve joint function.

The origins of chiropractic can be traced back to the late 19th century, when Daniel David Palmer, a magnetic healer, performed the first chiropractic adjustment on a deaf janitor. Palmer believed that the janitor's hearing loss was caused by a misalignment of his spine, and that by correcting the misalignment, he could restore his hearing. The janitor's hearing did indeed improve, and Palmer went on to develop chiropractic as a system of healing.

Chiropractic philosophy is based on the idea that the body has an innate ability to heal itself, and that this healing process can be facilitated by removing interference to the nervous system. Chiropractors believe that misalignments in the spine, known as vertebral subluxations, can interfere with the flow of nerve impulses and cause a variety of health problems.

Chiropractors use a holistic approach to healthcare, focusing not just on the specific symptoms that a patient presents with, but on the overall health and well-being of the individual. They take into account a patient's lifestyle, diet, and emotional state, as well as any physical factors that may be contributing to their condition.

Chiropractic treatment typically involves a series of adjustments, or manipulations, of the spine and other joints in the body. These adjustments are designed to improve joint function, reduce pain, and restore mobility. Chiropractors may also use a variety of other techniques, such as massage, stretching, and exercise therapy, to help their patients achieve optimal health.

Chiropractic has been shown to be effective in the treatment of a variety of musculoskeletal conditions, including back pain, neck pain, and headaches. It has also been used to treat other conditions, such as asthma, allergies, and digestive disorders, although the scientific evidence for these uses is less clear.

One of the key principles of chiropractic is the idea of the subluxation, or misalignment of the spine. Chiropractors believe that subluxations can interfere with the normal functioning of the nervous system, causing a variety of health problems. However, the concept of the subluxation is controversial, and there is no consensus within the medical community as to its validity.

Chiropractors are licensed healthcare professionals who have completed extensive training in the diagnosis and treatment of musculoskeletal disorders. They are regulated by state licensing boards, and must adhere to strict standards of professional conduct and ethics.

In addition to their formal training, many chiropractors continue to pursue ongoing education and professional development throughout their careers. This helps them stay up-to-date with the latest research and techniques in their field, and ensures that they are providing the best possible care to their patients.

Origins and history

Chiropractic is a popular form of alternative medicine that focuses on the diagnosis and treatment of musculoskeletal disorders, particularly those related to the spine. It is based on the principle that the body has the innate ability to heal itself, and that a properly functioning nervous system is essential to overall health and well-being. Chiropractic is rooted in a long history of healing practices, and its origins can be traced back to ancient civilizations.

The origins of chiropractic can be traced back to the ancient Greeks, who believed that good health was the result of a balance of the four bodily fluids, or "humors." The Greek physician Hippocrates, often called the "father of medicine," emphasized the importance of manual therapies, including spinal manipulation, in the treatment of illness and injury.

In the 19th century, a number of individuals began to explore the potential benefits of manual therapies for treating various health conditions. One of the pioneers in this field was a Canadian healer named Daniel David Palmer, who is considered the founder of modern chiropractic. In 1895, Palmer performed the first chiropractic adjustment on a patient who had been suffering from hearing loss, and the patient reported an improvement in his hearing as a result of the treatment.

Palmer's approach to chiropractic was based on the idea that misalignments of the spine, or "subluxations," can interfere with the proper functioning of the nervous system, leading to a wide range of health problems. He believed that by manipulating the spine to correct these subluxations, the body's natural healing processes could be activated, leading to improved health and well-being.

Over the years, chiropractic has evolved into a complex and multifaceted field, with a range of different techniques and approaches used by practitioners around the world. While spinal manipulation remains a central focus of chiropractic care, many chiropractors also incorporate other modalities, such as massage, exercise, and nutritional counseling, into their treatment plans.

Today, chiropractic is recognized as a legitimate form of healthcare in many countries around the world, and millions of people seek out chiropractic care every year for a wide range of health concerns. While there is still some controversy surrounding the safety and effectiveness of chiropractic care, many patients report significant improvements in their health and quality of life as a result of treatment. With its long and rich history, chiropractic is sure to continue evolving and adapting to meet the changing needs of patients in the years to come.

Philosophy and principles

Chiropractic is a form of alternative medicine that primarily focuses on diagnosing and treating musculoskeletal system disorders, especially spinal issues, through manual manipulation and adjustment of the spine. While chiropractic has become increasingly popular in recent years, it has been around for more than a century.

The philosophy and principles of chiropractic date back to the late 19th century, when Daniel David Palmer, a Canadian-born magnetic healer, made a significant discovery that would ultimately form the basis of the chiropractic practice. In 1895, he performed the first chiropractic adjustment on a patient named Harvey Lillard, who had lost his hearing 17 years prior. Palmer identified a misaligned vertebra in Lillard's spine and hypothesized that this could be the cause of his deafness. After realigning the vertebra through a series of manual manipulations, Lillard's hearing was restored.

This discovery led Palmer to develop a new approach to healing, which he named "chiropractic." He believed that the human body had an innate ability to heal itself and that any disruption to this process could lead to various illnesses and disorders. Chiropractic, therefore, aimed to restore the body's natural healing ability by removing any interference in the nervous system, which he believed was responsible for many health issues.

Chiropractic philosophy is rooted in the principle that the body has the ability to heal itself, given the right conditions. This principle, known as "vitalism," emphasizes the importance of maintaining a healthy nervous system, which is responsible for coordinating and controlling all body functions. Chiropractors believe that any misalignments or subluxations in the spine can disrupt the nervous system's functioning, leading to pain, discomfort, and other health issues.

Chiropractic principles also recognize the interconnectedness of the body, meaning that any issues in one part of the body can affect the functioning of other parts. Chiropractors, therefore, view the body as a holistic system, rather than just individual parts.

Chiropractors also believe that the body's structure, particularly the spine, plays a vital role in maintaining overall health and well-being. They believe that the spine is the center of the body and that any misalignments or subluxations can cause a range of health issues. As such, chiropractic treatments aim to realign and adjust the spine to restore optimal health and functioning.

Another key principle of chiropractic is the emphasis on natural, drug-free healing. Chiropractors believe that the body has the ability to heal itself naturally, and as such, they focus on providing non-invasive, drug-free treatments. Chiropractors also believe in the importance of lifestyle changes and patient education to promote overall health and prevent future health issues.

Chiropractic vs traditional medicine

Chiropractic is a form of alternative medicine that focuses on diagnosing and treating mechanical disorders of the musculoskeletal system, especially the spine. While chiropractors work within the healthcare industry, they often have different approaches to treatment than traditional medicine. Below we will explore the differences between chiropractic and traditional medicine.

Traditional medicine, also known as Western medicine or allopathic medicine, is a system of medicine that is based on the scientific method and has been taught in medical schools for over a century. Traditional medicine focuses on the diagnosis and treatment of disease, with an emphasis on the use of medication, surgery, and other invasive procedures. The primary goal of traditional medicine is to eliminate the disease or condition through intervention.

Chiropractic, on the other hand, is based on the principle that the body has an innate ability to heal itself. Chiropractors believe that mechanical disorders of the musculoskeletal system, particularly the spine, can interfere with the body's natural healing abilities. Chiropractors aim to restore the body's natural balance and function by addressing these mechanical disorders through a variety of manual therapies, including spinal manipulation, soft tissue manipulation, and stretching exercises.

One of the primary differences between chiropractic and traditional medicine is the approach to treatment. Traditional medicine often focuses on treating the symptoms of a disease or condition, rather than addressing the underlying cause. For example, if a patient presents with lower back pain, a traditional medical doctor may prescribe pain medication or recommend surgery. While these interventions may provide temporary relief, they do not address the root cause of the pain.

Chiropractors, on the other hand, seek to identify and address the underlying cause of a patient's pain or discomfort. They believe that spinal misalignments or other mechanical disorders can cause a wide range of symptoms, including pain, stiffness, and limited mobility. By identifying and correcting these mechanical disorders, chiropractors aim to restore the body's natural balance and function, thereby addressing the underlying cause of the patient's symptoms.

Another difference between chiropractic and traditional medicine is the use of diagnostic tools. Traditional medicine relies heavily on laboratory tests, imaging studies, and other diagnostic tools to identify and diagnose disease. Chiropractic, on the other hand, relies primarily on the chiropractor's physical examination and patient history to diagnose mechanical disorders of the musculoskeletal system. While imaging studies may be ordered if necessary, they are not typically the first line of diagnostic testing in chiropractic care.

Finally, there is a difference in the length of treatment between chiropractic and traditional medicine. Traditional medical treatments often involve a short course of medication or a single surgical intervention. Chiropractic care, on the other hand, often involves a series of treatments over an extended period. This is because chiropractors believe that the body's natural healing process takes time and that restoring the body's natural balance and function requires ongoing treatment and maintenance.

Chapter Two

The Spine and Nervous System

Chiropractic is a healthcare discipline that focuses on the musculoskeletal and nervous systems, with a particular emphasis on the spine. The spine and nervous system are intricately connected, and chiropractors work to optimize this connection to promote overall health and wellness. Below we will explore the relationship between the spine and nervous system and how chiropractic care can benefit both.

1. The spine is the main structural support for the body and is made up of 33 individual vertebrae. These vertebrae are divided into five regions: cervical (neck), thoracic (upper back), lumbar (lower back), sacral (pelvic), and coccygeal (tailbone). The spine not only provides support but also houses and protects the spinal cord, which is the main pathway for communication between the brain and the rest of the body.

The nervous system consists of the brain, spinal cord, and nerves that extend throughout the body. It is responsible for controlling and coordinating all of the body's functions, including movement, sensation, and organ function. The spinal cord acts as the main pathway for communication between the brain and the rest of the body. The spinal cord is protected by the vertebrae, which also provide support and stability for the body.

When there is a misalignment in the spine, it can disrupt the normal flow of information through the nervous system. This can lead to a wide range of health problems, including pain, muscle weakness, and organ dysfunction. Chiropractors believe that by restoring proper alignment and function to the spine, they can help to optimize the function of the nervous system and promote overall health and wellness.

Chiropractic adjustments, also known as spinal manipulations, are the primary method of treatment used by chiropractors. During an adjustment, the chiropractor will use their hands to apply a controlled force to a specific joint in the spine. This force helps to realign the joint, restore proper function, and alleviate pain and other symptoms.

In addition to spinal adjustments, chiropractors may also use a variety of other techniques to promote spinal health and optimize nervous system function. These techniques may include massage, stretching, exercise, and lifestyle counseling. Chiropractors may also work in conjunction with other healthcare professionals, such as physical therapists, to provide comprehensive care for their patients.

One of the primary benefits of chiropractic care is that it is a non-invasive, drug-free approach to healthcare. Chiropractors work to promote natural healing and encourage the body to function at its best. This can be especially beneficial for individuals who may be unable or unwilling to take medications or undergo invasive procedures.

Chiropractic care has been shown to be effective in treating a wide range of conditions, including back pain, neck pain, headaches, and sciatica. It has also been shown to be effective in treating conditions such as asthma, digestive issues, and menstrual problems, which may not seem to be related to spinal health at first glance. This is because the nervous system has an impact on all of the body's functions, and by promoting optimal nervous system function, chiropractors can help to improve overall health and wellness.

Anatomy and function

Chiropractic is a form of alternative medicine that is based on the idea that the body has an innate ability to heal itself, provided that the spine and nervous system are functioning properly. As such, chiropractors focus on the diagnosis and treatment of musculoskeletal disorders, particularly those affecting the spine. In order to understand the principles of chiropractic, it is important to have a basic understanding of the anatomy and function of the spine and nervous system.

1. The spine is composed of 33 individual vertebrae that are stacked on top of each other. The vertebrae are divided into five regions: cervical (neck), thoracic (upper back), lumbar (lower back), sacral (pelvis), and coccygeal (tailbone). The spine is not a straight line but rather it has natural curves that are important for maintaining proper posture and balance.

The primary function of the spine is to protect the spinal cord, which is a bundle of nerves that runs from the brain down through the spinal canal. The spinal cord serves as the main pathway for transmitting signals between the brain and the rest of the body. These signals control virtually all bodily functions, including movement, sensation, and organ function.

The spinal cord is also surrounded by cerebrospinal fluid, which helps to cushion it and protect it from injury. The nerves that branch off from the spinal cord exit the spine through small openings between the vertebrae, called intervertebral foramina.

2. The nervous system is composed of the brain, spinal cord, and nerves, and it is responsible for controlling all bodily functions. The nervous system is divided into two parts: the central nervous system (CNS) and the peripheral nervous system (PNS). The CNS consists of the brain and spinal cord, while the PNS consists of all the nerves that branch off from the CNS and extend throughout the body.

3. The PNS is further divided into two branches: the somatic nervous system and the autonomic nervous system. The somatic nervous system controls voluntary movements and sensation, while the autonomic nervous system controls involuntary bodily functions, such as heart rate, digestion, and breathing.

4. The autonomic nervous system is further divided into two branches: the sympathetic nervous system and the parasympathetic nervous system. The sympathetic nervous system is responsible for the body's "fight or flight" response to stress, while the parasympathetic nervous system is responsible for the body's "rest and digest" response to relaxation.

The spine and nervous system are intimately connected, and dysfunction in one can often lead to dysfunction in the other. For example, misalignments or subluxations in the spine can put pressure on the nerves that exit the spinal cord, causing pain, inflammation, and other symptoms. Conversely, dysfunction in the nervous system can lead to muscle tension, spasms, and other musculoskeletal problems.

Chiropractors use a variety of techniques to diagnose and treat musculoskeletal disorders, with a particular focus on the spine and nervous system. These techniques include spinal adjustments, massage, stretching, and exercise therapy. Spinal adjustments involve the application of gentle pressure to specific areas of the spine in order to realign the vertebrae and relieve pressure on the nerves. This can help to reduce pain, inflammation, and other symptoms, and improve overall bodily function.

In addition to treating musculoskeletal disorders, chiropractors also focus on maintaining overall health and wellness. They may offer advice on nutrition, exercise, stress management, and other lifestyle factors that can impact the health of the spine and nervous system. Chiropractors believe that by addressing these factors, they can help to prevent disease and promote optimal health and well-being.

The importance of spinal health

Chiropractic care is a type of alternative medicine that focuses on the diagnosis and treatment of neuromuscular disorders, particularly those affecting the spine. The spine plays a crucial role in the body, providing support and protection for the spinal cord, which is the main pathway for communication between the brain and the rest of the body. As such, maintaining spinal health is essential for overall physical and emotional well-being.

The spine is composed of 33 vertebrae, separated by intervertebral discs, which act as shock absorbers. The spine is also surrounded by a network of muscles, ligaments, and nerves, which work together to provide stability and movement. The spinal cord runs through the spinal canal, which is formed by the vertebrae, and is responsible for transmitting messages between the brain and the rest of the body.

When the spine is misaligned, it can cause interference with the nervous system, leading to a range of health problems. This is where chiropractic care comes in. Chiropractors use manual manipulation techniques to adjust the spine, restoring proper alignment and improving nerve function. This can help to alleviate pain, improve mobility, and enhance overall health and wellness.

Chiropractic care is based on the principle that the body has the innate ability to heal itself, and that the nervous system plays a key role in this process. When the spine is misaligned, it can cause interference with the nervous system, disrupting the body's natural healing mechanisms. By restoring proper alignment to the spine, chiropractors can help to remove this interference, allowing the body to heal itself.

Chiropractors use a variety of techniques to manipulate the spine, including spinal adjustments, spinal decompression, and soft tissue therapy. Spinal adjustments involve the application of controlled force to specific vertebrae, with the goal of restoring proper alignment and range of motion. Spinal decompression involves the use of traction to relieve pressure on the spine and intervertebral discs, while soft tissue therapy involves the use of massage and other techniques to loosen tight muscles and improve circulation.

Maintaining spinal health is essential for overall physical and emotional well-being. In addition to chiropractic care, there are several steps you can take to support spinal health. These include maintaining good posture, practicing proper lifting techniques, and engaging in regular exercise. You should also avoid smoking and excessive alcohol consumption, as these can contribute to spinal degeneration.

Common spinal issues and conditions

Chiropractic is a holistic approach to healthcare that focuses on the spine and nervous system, and its goal is to promote overall wellness and optimal body function. Chiropractors believe that the body has a natural ability to heal itself, and they use various techniques to help restore the body's natural balance and function. The spine is a critical component of this system, and any misalignments or issues with the spine can lead to a wide range of health problems. Below we will explore some common spinal issues and conditions that can benefit from chiropractic care.

One of the most common spinal issues that chiropractors encounter is spinal misalignment, also known as subluxation. A subluxation occurs when one or more of the vertebrae in the spine become misaligned or move out of their proper position. This can put pressure on the surrounding nerves, causing pain and discomfort. Symptoms of subluxation can vary widely, and may include pain, stiffness, muscle weakness, numbness, tingling, and even digestive problems or headaches. Chiropractors use spinal adjustments to correct subluxations, which involves gentle manipulations of the spine to help realign the vertebrae and relieve pressure on the nerves. This can provide significant pain relief and improve overall spinal health.

Another common spinal issue is herniated discs, which occur when the soft, jelly-like material inside the discs that cushion the vertebrae leaks out and puts pressure on the surrounding nerves. This can cause pain, numbness, and tingling in the affected area, and may even lead to weakness or paralysis in severe cases. Chiropractic care can be an effective treatment for herniated discs, as chiropractors can use spinal adjustments to relieve pressure on the affected nerves and help the discs heal naturally. They may also use other techniques, such as traction or massage therapy, to promote healing and reduce inflammation in the affected area.

Spinal stenosis is another common spinal condition that can benefit from chiropractic care. Spinal stenosis occurs when the spaces within the spine become narrowed, putting pressure on the nerves and causing pain and discomfort. This can be caused by a variety of factors, including arthritis, disc degeneration, or injury. Chiropractic care can be an effective treatment for spinal stenosis, as chiropractors can use gentle spinal adjustments to help realign the vertebrae and relieve pressure on the nerves. They may also use other techniques, such as stretching or massage therapy, to help alleviate pain and improve range of motion in the affected area.

Sciatica is a common condition that affects the sciatic nerve, which runs from the lower back down to the legs. When the sciatic nerve becomes compressed or irritated, it can cause pain, numbness, and tingling in the affected area. Chiropractic care can be an effective treatment for sciatica, as chiropractors can use spinal adjustments to help relieve pressure on the sciatic nerve and reduce inflammation in the affected area. They may also use other techniques, such as massage or stretching, to help alleviate pain and improve overall mobility.

Chapter Three

Chiropractic Techniques

Chiropractic techniques are used to treat a variety of spinal and musculoskeletal conditions. These techniques involve manual adjustments of the spine, joints, and soft tissues to improve alignment, reduce pain, and restore normal function. There are several different chiropractic techniques that are used depending on the patient's condition and preferences.

One common technique is called the diversified technique. This technique involves the chiropractor using their hands to apply a quick, high-velocity thrust to a joint that is restricted in its movement. The goal of this technique is to restore normal motion and alignment to the joint, and to reduce pain and inflammation.

Another technique is the Gonstead technique. This technique involves the chiropractor using a combination of palpation, X-rays, and other diagnostic tools to identify the specific problem areas in the spine. The chiropractor then uses manual adjustments to restore proper alignment and function to the affected areas.

The activator technique is another commonly used chiropractic technique. This technique uses a small handheld instrument that delivers a gentle, low-force thrust to the affected area. This technique is often preferred by patients who are uncomfortable with the more forceful manual adjustments used in other techniques.

The Thompson technique is another popular chiropractic technique. This technique uses a specialized table that drops slightly when pressure is applied to the patient's spine. This drop in the table allows the chiropractor to apply a gentle, low-force adjustment to the affected area.

In addition to these specific techniques, chiropractors may also use massage, stretching, and other manual therapies to improve the patient's overall condition. Chiropractors may also provide patients with advice on lifestyle changes, exercise, and nutrition to support the body's natural healing process.

It is important to note that while chiropractic techniques are generally safe, there are some risks and potential side effects associated with these treatments. These risks can include soreness or stiffness after treatment, headaches, and in rare cases, more serious complications such as stroke or nerve damage. It is important for patients to discuss any potential risks with their chiropractor before starting treatment.

Spinal manipulation

Spinal manipulation is a chiropractic technique that is used to relieve pain, reduce inflammation, and improve the overall function of the body. It is a non-invasive and drug-free approach to healthcare that is safe for people of all ages. Below we will explore what spinal manipulation is, how it works, and the benefits of this chiropractic technique.

Spinal manipulation is a manual therapy that involves the application of force to the spine using various techniques. This force is applied to specific areas of the spine that are not moving correctly or are out of alignment. By applying this force, chiropractors aim to restore the proper movement and alignment of the spine, which can help to reduce pain and inflammation in the affected area.

One of the most common techniques used in spinal manipulation is called high-velocity low-amplitude (HVLA) thrust. This technique involves a quick and precise thrust to the spine, which is often accompanied by an audible popping sound. This sound is caused by the release of gas bubbles that have built up in the joints of the spine.

Another technique used in spinal manipulation is called flexion-distraction. This technique involves the use of a specially designed table that allows the chiropractor to gently stretch and flex the spine. This technique is often used to treat conditions such as herniated discs and sciatica.

Spinal manipulation works by restoring the proper movement and alignment of the spine. When the spine is not moving correctly or is out of alignment, it can cause pressure on the nerves that run through the spine. This pressure can lead to pain, inflammation, and a host of other health issues.

By restoring the proper movement and alignment of the spine, chiropractors aim to reduce pressure on the nerves and promote healing in the affected area. This can lead to a reduction in pain, inflammation, and other symptoms associated with spinal issues.

One of the main benefits of spinal manipulation is that it is a non-invasive and drug-free approach to healthcare. Unlike surgery or medication, spinal manipulation does not involve any incisions or the use of drugs. This makes it a safe and effective option for people of all ages who are looking for a natural approach to healthcare.

Another benefit of spinal manipulation is that it can be used to treat a wide range of conditions. Spinal manipulation is often used to treat conditions such as back pain, neck pain, headaches, and sciatica. It can also be used to treat conditions such as carpal tunnel syndrome, fibromyalgia, and sports injuries.

In addition to its benefits for the treatment of specific conditions, spinal manipulation can also be used to improve overall health and wellness. By restoring the proper movement and alignment of the spine, chiropractors can help to improve the function of the nervous system, which is essential for overall health and wellness.

Mobilization

Chiropractic is a healthcare profession that focuses on the diagnosis, treatment, and prevention of musculoskeletal and nervous system disorders. The practice of chiropractic involves the use of manual therapies, including spinal manipulation and mobilization, to improve joint function and relieve pain. Mobilization is a technique used in chiropractic care to treat a variety of musculoskeletal conditions.

Mobilization is a gentle technique that involves the passive movement of a joint through its range of motion. During mobilization, a chiropractor uses manual pressure to move the joint within its normal anatomical limits. The goal of mobilization is to restore normal joint function, reduce pain, and improve the patient's overall mobility. Mobilization is typically used in conjunction with other chiropractic techniques, such as spinal manipulation and soft tissue therapies.

Mobilization can be used to treat a wide range of musculoskeletal conditions, including back pain, neck pain, shoulder pain, and hip pain. It is also used to treat conditions such as arthritis, bursitis, and tendonitis. Mobilization is often used as a gentle alternative to spinal manipulation, which may not be appropriate for all patients.

Mobilization is performed in a series of gentle, rhythmic movements that gradually increase in intensity. The chiropractor may also use various other techniques to enhance the effectiveness of the mobilization, such as stretching, massage, or hot and cold therapy. The patient is usually positioned lying down or sitting, and the chiropractor will use their hands or a specialized tool to apply the necessary pressure to the joint.

Mobilization is generally safe and well-tolerated by most patients. However, as with any medical treatment, there are potential risks and side effects associated with mobilization. These may include soreness, stiffness, and temporary aggravation of the symptoms. Patients with certain conditions, such as osteoporosis or arthritis, may be at a higher risk for complications from mobilization, and should discuss their individual risks with their chiropractor.

Chiropractors use a variety of diagnostic and treatment techniques to address musculoskeletal disorders. In addition to mobilization, chiropractors may use other manual therapies, such as spinal manipulation and soft tissue therapies, to improve joint function and reduce pain. They may also incorporate other techniques into their treatment plans, such as exercises, dietary changes, and lifestyle modifications. Chiropractic care is often used in conjunction with traditional medical care to provide a holistic approach to healthcare.

Soft tissue techniques

Chiropractic is a healthcare discipline that focuses on the diagnosis and treatment of musculoskeletal and nervous system disorders. Soft tissue techniques are one of the chiropractic techniques used to treat soft tissue injuries. Soft tissue refers to the muscle, tendons, ligaments, and fascia that support and connect the body's structure.

Soft tissue techniques used in chiropractic care are manual therapies used to relieve pain and restore normal function. These techniques work by applying pressure, tension, or movement to the affected areas to reduce tension, adhesions, and pain.

One of the most common soft tissue techniques used in chiropractic is called myofascial release. This technique is used to release tension and adhesions in the fascia, which is the connective tissue that surrounds and supports muscles, bones, and organs. Myofascial release involves applying sustained pressure to the affected area, followed by a gentle stretching motion.

Another soft tissue technique used in chiropractic is trigger point therapy. Trigger points are localized areas of tightness and tenderness in the muscle tissue. Trigger point therapy involves applying pressure to these areas to release tension and reduce pain.

Graston Technique is another soft tissue technique that is commonly used in chiropractic care. This technique involves the use of specially designed instruments to break up scar tissue and adhesions in the soft tissues.

Active Release Technique (ART) is another soft tissue technique used in chiropractic care. This technique involves the use of specific movements and manual pressure to break up scar tissue and adhesions in the muscles and other soft tissues.

In addition to these techniques, chiropractors may also use heat and cold therapy, ultrasound, and electrical stimulation to treat soft tissue injuries. These treatments work by increasing blood flow, reducing inflammation, and promoting healing.

Soft tissue techniques used in chiropractic care can be highly effective in treating a wide range of conditions, including back pain, neck pain, and headaches. These techniques can also be used to treat sports injuries, carpal tunnel syndrome, and other soft tissue injuries.

Chiropractors often combine soft tissue techniques with other chiropractic techniques, such as spinal adjustments, to provide a comprehensive approach to care. By addressing both the soft tissue and structural components of a condition, chiropractors can help patients achieve optimal health and wellness.

Chapter Four

Assessment and Diagnosis

Chiropractors are healthcare professionals who focus on the diagnosis and treatment of musculoskeletal and nervous system disorders, with a particular emphasis on the spine. In order to develop effective treatment plans, chiropractors must first conduct thorough assessments and make accurate diagnoses. Below we will explore the assessment and diagnosis process in chiropractic care.

The assessment process typically begins with a detailed health history and physical examination. The chiropractor will ask the patient about their symptoms, medical history, lifestyle, and other relevant information. They will also perform a physical examination, which may include range of motion tests, palpation of the spine and other areas of the body, and neurological tests.

In addition to the health history and physical exam, chiropractors may use diagnostic imaging tests to further evaluate the patient's condition. X-rays, CT scans, and MRI scans can provide detailed images of the spine and surrounding tissues, which can help the chiropractor identify any structural abnormalities or injuries.

Once the assessment is complete, the chiropractor will use the information gathered to make a diagnosis. Chiropractors use a variety of diagnostic tools and techniques to identify the root cause of the patient's symptoms. They may use manual palpation to locate areas of restricted movement or tenderness, or they may use diagnostic imaging to evaluate the alignment of the spine and surrounding structures.

Chiropractors may also use a technique known as motion palpation, which involves feeling for areas of the spine that are not moving properly. This can help identify joint dysfunction or other musculoskeletal issues that may be contributing to the patient's symptoms.

In addition to evaluating the spine, chiropractors may also assess other areas of the body that may be contributing to the patient's condition. For example, if the patient is experiencing headaches, the chiropractor may examine the muscles and joints in the neck to determine if there is any tension or misalignment that could be causing the headaches.

Once a diagnosis has been made, the chiropractor will work with the patient to develop a personalized treatment plan. Treatment may involve a combination of manual therapies, such as spinal manipulation and soft tissue techniques, as well as exercises and lifestyle modifications to support overall health and wellbeing.

In some cases, chiropractors may refer patients to other healthcare providers for further evaluation or treatment. For example, if the patient is experiencing back pain that is caused by a herniated disc, the chiropractor may refer the patient to a spine specialist for further evaluation and possible surgical intervention.

It is important to note that chiropractic care is not appropriate for all conditions. Chiropractors are trained to recognize when a patient's symptoms may be caused by an underlying medical condition that requires treatment from a different type of healthcare provider. In these cases, the chiropractor will work with the patient to ensure that they receive the appropriate care.

Patient history

Chiropractic care is a healthcare profession that focuses on the diagnosis, treatment, and prevention of mechanical disorders of the musculoskeletal system, particularly the spine. As with any healthcare profession, chiropractors gather information about their patients' medical history and overall health status to help determine an accurate diagnosis and create a customized treatment plan. Patient history is an essential part of chiropractic care because it helps chiropractors understand their patients' unique health needs and identify any underlying conditions that may affect their care.

When a patient comes in for chiropractic care, the chiropractor will typically begin by gathering a comprehensive medical history. This includes asking the patient about their current symptoms, past medical history, family history, lifestyle habits, and any medications or supplements they are currently taking. The chiropractor may also ask the patient about their diet, exercise routine, and work or recreational activities that may contribute to their symptoms.

By gathering this information, chiropractors can better understand their patients' overall health and identify any potential risk factors or underlying conditions that may affect their care. For example, if a patient has a family history of heart disease, the chiropractor may take this into account when creating a treatment plan that includes cardiovascular exercise or dietary changes.

Another important part of the patient history is information about the patient's current symptoms. Chiropractors will ask about the location, duration, and severity of the patient's pain or discomfort, as well as any other symptoms they may be experiencing, such as numbness, tingling, or weakness. This information can help the chiropractor identify the specific structures that may be causing the patient's symptoms and determine the best course of treatment.

In addition to gathering a medical history, chiropractors may also perform a physical examination to further assess the patient's condition. This may include testing the patient's reflexes, range of motion, and strength, as well as conducting orthopedic and neurological tests to help identify any underlying conditions.

By combining the information gathered from the patient history and physical examination, chiropractors can make an accurate diagnosis and create a customized treatment plan that addresses the patient's specific health needs. This may include chiropractic adjustments, soft tissue therapy, exercise recommendations, and lifestyle changes, among other interventions.

It is important to note that patient history is an ongoing process throughout the course of chiropractic care. Chiropractors will continue to gather information about their patients' symptoms, progress, and overall health status to ensure that they are receiving the most effective and appropriate care possible. This may include regular follow-up appointments, additional testing or imaging, or referrals to other healthcare providers as needed.

Physical examination

Chiropractic is a healthcare profession that focuses on the diagnosis and treatment of musculoskeletal and nervous system disorders, with a particular emphasis on the spine. Chiropractors use a variety of techniques to help relieve pain and improve function, including spinal manipulation, mobilization, and soft tissue techniques. However, before any treatment can be provided, a thorough assessment and diagnosis must be conducted.

The initial step in the assessment process for chiropractors is obtaining a detailed patient history. This involves gathering information on the patient's current complaint, as well as any previous medical conditions, surgeries, or injuries that may be relevant to their current condition. It is also important to obtain information about the patient's lifestyle, such as their occupation, hobbies, and exercise habits, as these may have an impact on their condition.

Next, a physical examination is conducted to assess the patient's musculoskeletal and nervous system. This typically involves a variety of tests and procedures, including range of motion assessments, muscle strength testing, reflex testing, and sensory testing. The chiropractor may also use imaging studies such as X-rays or MRIs to get a better understanding of the patient's condition.

During the physical examination, the chiropractor will also assess the patient's spinal alignment and joint mobility. They will use palpation techniques to identify areas of tenderness, swelling, or other abnormalities. This information is used to develop a treatment plan that is tailored to the patient's specific needs.

In some cases, the chiropractor may refer the patient for further diagnostic testing or consultation with another healthcare provider. This is particularly true if the patient's condition is complex or requires additional medical intervention.

It is important to note that chiropractic care is not appropriate for all patients. Patients with certain medical conditions, such as osteoporosis or spinal fractures, may not be candidates for spinal manipulation or other chiropractic techniques. Additionally, some patients may experience adverse reactions to chiropractic care, such as temporary soreness or fatigue.

These risks and contraindications are carefully evaluated during the assessment and diagnosis process.

Diagnostic imaging

Chiropractic care is a non-invasive and drug-free approach to treating musculoskeletal conditions, which focuses on the spine and nervous system. Chiropractors use a variety of diagnostic techniques to determine the underlying cause of a patient's symptoms. One of the most commonly used diagnostic tools in chiropractic care is diagnostic imaging.

Diagnostic imaging is the process of creating visual representations of the body's internal structures. This is done to identify any abnormalities or injuries that may be causing a patient's pain or discomfort. In chiropractic care, there are several types of diagnostic imaging techniques that may be used.

X-rays are a commonly used form of diagnostic imaging in chiropractic care. An X-ray machine emits a small amount of radiation that passes through the body and is absorbed by bones and other tissues to varying degrees. This produces a black and white image of the internal structures, which can be used to identify fractures, misalignments, or other abnormalities.

Magnetic resonance imaging (MRI) is another diagnostic imaging technique that is used in chiropractic care. Unlike X-rays, MRI uses a strong magnetic field and radio waves to create detailed images of the body's internal structures. This can help chiropractors to identify soft tissue injuries, such as herniated discs, and determine the extent of the damage.

Computed tomography (CT) scans are also used in chiropractic care. CT scans use a series of X-rays to create a three-dimensional image of the body's internal structures. This can be used to identify fractures, tumors, or other abnormalities that may not be visible on X-rays alone.

Ultrasound is another diagnostic imaging technique that is used in chiropractic care. This involves using high-frequency sound waves to create images of the body's internal structures. Ultrasound is often used to examine soft tissues, such as muscles and tendons, and can be useful in identifying injuries such as sprains or strains.

Chiropractors may also use thermography, which uses infrared technology to create images of the body's temperature patterns. This can be useful in identifying areas of inflammation, which can be indicative of an underlying injury or condition.

In addition to diagnostic imaging, chiropractors may also use other diagnostic tools such as physical exams, patient history, and laboratory tests to help determine the underlying cause of a patient's symptoms.

It is important to note that while diagnostic imaging can be a valuable tool in chiropractic care, it is not always necessary. Chiropractors will only recommend diagnostic imaging if it is necessary to accurately diagnose and treat a patient's condition. Additionally, chiropractors will always take precautions to minimize a patient's exposure to radiation when using X-rays.

Chapter Five

Chiropractic Care for Various Conditions

Chiropractic care is a form of alternative medicine that focuses on the diagnosis and treatment of musculoskeletal disorders, particularly those affecting the spine. Chiropractic care is a non-invasive and drug-free approach to healing that aims to improve overall health and well-being.

Chiropractic care can be used to treat a wide range of conditions, including back pain, neck pain, headaches, and other musculoskeletal disorders. Here are some of the most common conditions that chiropractors can help to treat.

1. Back Pain: Chiropractors are perhaps best known for their ability to treat back pain. This can include acute back pain caused by an injury or chronic back pain caused by degenerative conditions such as arthritis. Chiropractors use a variety of techniques to help alleviate back pain, including spinal adjustments, mobilization, and soft tissue therapies.

2. Neck Pain: Chiropractic care can also be very effective for treating neck pain. Neck pain can be caused by a variety of factors, including poor posture, whiplash, and degenerative conditions such as arthritis. Chiropractors use a range of techniques to help alleviate neck pain, including spinal adjustments and soft tissue therapies.

3. Headaches: Chiropractic care can be an effective treatment for tension headaches and migraines. Many headaches are caused by tension in the

neck and shoulders, and chiropractors can help to alleviate this tension through spinal adjustments and soft tissue therapies.

4. Sciatica: Sciatica is a condition characterized by pain, numbness, and tingling in the lower back and legs. Chiropractors can help to alleviate sciatica by using a combination of spinal adjustments and soft tissue therapies.

5. Sports Injuries: Chiropractic care can be very effective for treating sports injuries such as sprains, strains, and joint pain. Chiropractors can use a range of techniques to help reduce inflammation and promote healing, including spinal adjustments and soft tissue therapies.

6. Carpal Tunnel Syndrome: Carpal tunnel syndrome is a condition characterized by pain and numbness in the hands and wrists. Chiropractors can help to alleviate carpal tunnel syndrome by using a combination of spinal adjustments and soft tissue therapies.

7. Fibromyalgia: Fibromyalgia is a chronic condition characterized by widespread pain, fatigue, and sleep disturbances. Chiropractors can help to alleviate the pain associated with fibromyalgia by using a range of techniques, including spinal adjustments and soft tissue therapies.

8. Arthritis: Arthritis is a degenerative condition characterized by pain and inflammation in the joints. Chiropractic care can be effective for alleviating the pain associated with arthritis, particularly in the spine and neck.

9. Pregnancy-related back pain: Pregnancy can cause significant changes to a woman's body, including back pain. Chiropractic care can help to alleviate pregnancy-related back pain by using gentle techniques that are safe for both the mother and the unborn child.

10. Digestive issues: Chiropractic care can also be effective for alleviating digestive issues such as irritable bowel syndrome (IBS). Chiropractors can

use a range of techniques to help improve digestion and reduce inflammation in the gut.

Back pain

Chiropractic care is a popular form of alternative medicine that focuses on the spine and nervous system. One of the most common reasons why patients seek out chiropractic care is to address back pain. Below we will explore the various causes of back pain, how chiropractic care can help alleviate it, and what to expect during a chiropractic appointment.

Back pain can be caused by a variety of factors, including poor posture, muscle strain, injuries, and spinal misalignments. Chiropractors are trained to diagnose the root cause of a patient's back pain and develop an individualized treatment plan that may include spinal adjustments, soft tissue therapies, and exercise recommendations.

Spinal adjustments are a key component of chiropractic care for back pain. During a spinal adjustment, the chiropractor uses their hands or a specialized instrument to apply a controlled force to a specific joint in the spine. This helps to restore proper alignment and range of motion, reducing pressure on surrounding nerves and muscles.

Soft tissue therapies, such as massage and stretching, can also be used to complement spinal adjustments. These techniques help to relieve tension in the muscles and improve flexibility, which can further reduce pain and discomfort.

Exercise is another important aspect of chiropractic care for back pain. Chiropractors may recommend specific exercises or stretches to help strengthen the muscles that support the spine, improve posture, and prevent future injuries.

Chiropractic care can be effective for a wide range of back pain conditions, including:

1. Lower back pain: The lower back is a common area for pain and discomfort due to its large range of motion and weight-bearing responsibilities. Chiropractic adjustments and soft tissue therapies can help alleviate pain and improve mobility in the lower back.

2. Herniated or bulging discs: When a disc in the spine becomes herniated or bulges out of place, it can put pressure on nearby nerves, causing pain and discomfort. Chiropractic adjustments can help to alleviate this pressure and reduce pain.

3. Sciatica: Sciatica is a condition in which the sciatic nerve, which runs from the lower back down to the legs, becomes irritated or compressed. Chiropractic adjustments can help to reduce pressure on the sciatic nerve, reducing pain and discomfort.

4. Scoliosis: Scoliosis is a curvature of the spine that can cause back pain and other health issues. Chiropractic care can help to reduce the severity of the curve and alleviate pain and discomfort.

5. Spinal stenosis: Spinal stenosis is a condition in which the spinal canal narrows, putting pressure on the spinal cord and nerves. Chiropractic adjustments can help to relieve this pressure and reduce pain.

During a chiropractic appointment for back pain, the chiropractor will typically begin with a thorough physical examination and medical history review. They may also order diagnostic imaging, such as X-rays or MRI scans, to help identify any underlying issues.

Based on their findings, the chiropractor will develop a customized treatment plan that may include spinal adjustments, soft tissue therapies, and exercise recommendations. Treatment frequency and duration will depend on the severity of the back pain and the individual patient's needs.

Neck pain

Chiropractic is a form of alternative medicine that focuses on the diagnosis and treatment of musculoskeletal disorders, with a particular emphasis on the spine. Neck pain is a common condition that chiropractors often encounter, and chiropractic care can be an effective treatment option for this issue.

The neck, also known as the cervical spine, is made up of seven vertebrae and is responsible for supporting the weight of the head and allowing for movement. Neck pain can be caused by a variety of factors, including poor posture, injury, and underlying medical conditions.

Chiropractic care for neck pain typically involves a combination of manual therapy techniques, such as spinal manipulation and mobilization, as well as exercises and lifestyle modifications to address contributing factors.

Spinal manipulation, also known as an adjustment, involves the application of a controlled force to a joint in the spine in order to improve its function and reduce pain. This technique is often accompanied by a popping or cracking sound, which is the result of a release of gas bubbles from the joint. While some people may find this sound alarming, it is typically not painful and is considered a normal part of the adjustment process.

Mobilization is a gentler form of manual therapy that involves the application of low-force techniques to gradually move a joint through its range of motion. This technique may be used for patients who are uncomfortable with or unable to tolerate spinal manipulation.

In addition to manual therapy techniques, chiropractors may also recommend exercises and stretches to help improve range of motion, reduce pain, and prevent future injuries. Lifestyle modifications, such as improving posture and avoiding activities that exacerbate symptoms, may also be recommended.

Chiropractic care for neck pain has been shown to be effective in reducing pain and improving function. A 2017 systematic review of 26 randomized controlled trials found that spinal manipulation was associated with a significant reduction in neck pain compared to other interventions, such as exercise or medication. Another study published in the Journal of Manipulative and Physiological Therapeutics found that a combination of spinal manipulation and exercises was effective in reducing pain and improving function in patients with chronic neck pain.

It is important to note that while chiropractic care can be an effective treatment option for neck pain, it may not be appropriate for all patients. Certain medical conditions, such as spinal cord compression or infection, may require more invasive treatments, and patients with a history of neck surgery or trauma may need to be treated with extra caution.

Headaches and migraines

Chiropractic care has been found to be an effective treatment for various conditions, including headaches and migraines. Headaches can be debilitating, causing pain and discomfort that disrupts daily life. Chiropractors are trained to assess and diagnose the underlying causes of headaches and provide treatment to alleviate the symptoms.

There are various types of headaches, but the most common types are tension headaches and migraines. Tension headaches are caused by muscle tension in the neck and head. Migraines, on the other hand, are a neurological condition characterized by severe headaches, often accompanied by other symptoms such as nausea, vomiting, and sensitivity to light and sound.

Chiropractic care for tension headaches usually involves spinal adjustments to relieve tension in the neck and head muscles. The chiropractor will also evaluate the patient's posture and lifestyle habits, such as sleep position and computer use, to identify potential triggers for tension headaches. They may also recommend exercises or stretches to help prevent future tension headaches.

For migraines, chiropractic care focuses on addressing the underlying neurological issues. The chiropractor may use spinal adjustments, massage therapy, or other techniques to improve blood flow to the brain and reduce nerve irritation. Additionally, they may recommend dietary changes or supplements to address potential triggers such as food sensitivities or nutritional deficiencies.

Research has shown that chiropractic care can be effective in reducing the frequency and severity of both tension headaches and migraines. A study published in the Journal of Manipulative and Physiological Therapeutics found that patients who received chiropractic care experienced significant reductions in the number of migraines they experienced per month, as well as reduced pain intensity.

Another study published in the European Journal of Neurology found that chiropractic care was effective in reducing the frequency of tension headaches, as well as the intensity of the pain associated with them. The study found that patients who received chiropractic care experienced significant reductions in headache frequency, intensity, and duration compared to those who did not receive chiropractic care.

Chiropractic care is often used in conjunction with other treatments for headaches and migraines, such as medication or relaxation techniques. Many patients find that chiropractic care is a safe and effective alternative to medication, which can have side effects or be ineffective for some individuals.

In addition to spinal adjustments and other physical therapies, chiropractors may also provide lifestyle advice to help prevent headaches and migraines. This may include recommendations for exercise, stress management techniques, and dietary changes.

It is important for individuals experiencing headaches or migraines to seek professional medical advice to determine the underlying cause and appropriate treatment plan. Chiropractic care can be a valuable component of a comprehensive treatment plan for headache and migraine sufferers, offering safe and effective relief from pain and discomfort.

Sports injuries

Chiropractic care can be beneficial for athletes and those who engage in regular physical activity. Sports injuries are common and can range from minor sprains and strains to more serious injuries such as fractures or dislocations. Chiropractors can help athletes recover from injuries, prevent future injuries, and improve overall athletic performance.

Chiropractors use a holistic approach to sports injury treatment, taking into account the athlete's individual needs and goals. They use a combination of techniques, including spinal adjustments, soft tissue therapy, and exercise rehabilitation, to help athletes recover from injuries and improve their overall function and performance.

One of the most common sports injuries is a sprain or strain, which occurs when a ligament or muscle is stretched or torn. Chiropractic care can be effective in treating these injuries by using soft tissue techniques to reduce inflammation and improve circulation to the injured area. Chiropractors can also use spinal adjustments to realign the spine and joints, reducing pain and restoring proper function.

Another common sports injury is a herniated disc, which occurs when the soft, gel-like center of a spinal disc protrudes through a tear in the outer layer. Chiropractors can use spinal adjustments to realign the spine and relieve pressure on the affected disc, reducing pain and improving mobility.

Concussions are also a common sports injury, particularly in contact sports such as football or hockey. Chiropractors can work with athletes to develop a safe and effective return-to-play plan following a concussion, helping them to avoid long-term complications such as post-concussion syndrome.

Chiropractors can also help athletes prevent injuries by identifying areas of weakness or imbalances in the body and developing a personalized exercise and stretching program to address these issues. By improving overall function and reducing the risk of injury, chiropractic care can help athletes stay healthy and perform at their best.

In addition to treating specific sports injuries, chiropractic care can also be used to improve overall athletic performance. By improving joint mobility and muscle flexibility, chiropractors can help athletes move more efficiently and with less effort, allowing them to perform at a higher level. Chiropractors can also provide advice on nutrition and hydration, helping athletes to fuel their bodies for optimal performance.

It is important for athletes to seek treatment for sports injuries as soon as possible to prevent further damage and ensure a faster recovery. Chiropractic care can provide effective and non-invasive treatment options for a wide range of sports injuries, helping athletes to get back in the game as quickly and safely as possible.

Chapter Six

Chiropractic and Pediatrics

Chiropractic is a form of alternative medicine that focuses on the diagnosis and treatment of mechanical disorders of the musculoskeletal system, especially the spine. While chiropractic care is often associated with adults, it is also becoming increasingly popular among pediatric populations.

The principles of chiropractic care for children are similar to those for adults, but there are important differences. Pediatric chiropractic care requires a deep understanding of a child's physical and emotional development. Chiropractors who specialize in pediatric care use gentle techniques that are appropriate for children and avoid aggressive manipulation.

There are a number of reasons why parents may seek chiropractic care for their children. One of the most common reasons is to address issues related to the musculoskeletal system. These can include problems with posture, joint mobility, and flexibility. Children who participate in sports may also experience injuries that can be effectively treated through chiropractic care.

Chiropractic care can also be beneficial for children with chronic conditions such as asthma, allergies, and ear infections. Chiropractors believe that these conditions are related to dysfunction in the nervous system and that chiropractic adjustments can help to restore proper nerve function, allowing the body to heal itself.

Another area where chiropractic care may be beneficial for children is in the treatment of behavioral and developmental disorders. Many children with these conditions have difficulty with coordination and balance, which can be improved through chiropractic care. Chiropractors who specialize in pediatric care may also be able to provide counseling and other services to help children with these conditions.

Parents who are interested in seeking chiropractic care for their children should first consult with their pediatrician. The pediatrician can provide guidance on whether chiropractic care is appropriate for their child and can refer them to a qualified chiropractor who specializes in pediatric care.

Once a child is under the care of a chiropractor, the chiropractor will perform a thorough evaluation to identify any areas of concern. They will then develop a treatment plan that is appropriate for the child's age and physical condition. Treatment may include gentle adjustments to the spine, as well as exercises and other therapies designed to improve mobility and flexibility.

Chiropractic care for children is generally safe and effective when provided by a qualified chiropractor who specializes in pediatric care. However, as with any medical treatment, there are risks involved. Parents should always discuss the risks and benefits of chiropractic care with their pediatrician and chiropractor before beginning treatment.

Benefits for children

Chiropractic is a form of complementary and alternative medicine that has become increasingly popular in recent years. While it was traditionally thought of as a therapy for adults, more and more parents are seeking chiropractic care for their children as well. Chiropractors who work with children use gentle techniques to help improve their spinal alignment and promote overall wellness.

There are many benefits to chiropractic care for children. One of the most important is that it can help with the development of the nervous system. The spine is the backbone of the nervous system, and any misalignments can disrupt the way that signals are transmitted between the brain and the body. By ensuring proper spinal alignment, chiropractors can help children's nervous systems function properly, which can improve their overall health and well-being.

Chiropractic care can also help children who have chronic conditions or injuries. For example, children who suffer from asthma or allergies may benefit from chiropractic adjustments that help to improve their breathing. Similarly, children who participate in sports or other physical activities may be more prone to injuries, and chiropractic adjustments can help to improve their musculoskeletal health and reduce the risk of injury.

Another benefit of chiropractic care for children is that it can help with behavioral and emotional issues. Many children experience stress, anxiety, or even depression at some point in their lives. Chiropractic adjustments can help to reduce tension and promote relaxation, which can in turn help to reduce the symptoms of these conditions.

One of the unique aspects of chiropractic care for children is that it is generally very gentle and non-invasive. Unlike some other medical procedures, chiropractic adjustments do not involve any drugs or surgery. Instead, chiropractors use manual manipulation of the spine to help improve alignment and reduce tension. This means that children who receive chiropractic care are at very low risk of experiencing any negative side effects.

When working with children, chiropractors use different techniques than they do with adults. Children's spines are still developing, so chiropractors must use extra care to avoid causing any harm. They also tend to use gentler techniques, such as light pressure or massage, rather than the more forceful adjustments that are commonly used on adults.

In order to receive chiropractic care, children typically need to undergo a thorough evaluation. This may involve a physical exam, x-rays, and other tests to determine the nature and severity of any underlying issues. Chiropractors will also typically take into account the child's age, weight, and overall health when developing a treatment plan.

In general, children can benefit from chiropractic care in many of the same ways that adults can. By improving spinal alignment and reducing tension, chiropractors can help to improve children's overall health and wellness. Whether a child is dealing with chronic health issues or simply needs help managing stress and anxiety, chiropractic care can be a safe and effective option.

Adjusting techniques for young patients

Chiropractic is a non-invasive and drug-free approach to healthcare that focuses on the body's musculoskeletal system, particularly the spine, and how it affects the overall health of an individual. While commonly associated with adult patients, chiropractic care can also be beneficial for children. In fact, some chiropractors specialize in pediatric chiropractic care and receive additional training to provide safe and effective adjustments for young patients.

One of the main benefits of chiropractic care for children is that it can help improve their overall health and well-being. Adjustments can help to correct spinal misalignments, which can lead to a variety of health issues, including colic, ear infections, asthma, and ADHD. By correcting these misalignments, chiropractors can help to restore proper function to the nervous system and improve the body's natural healing abilities.

When it comes to adjusting techniques for young patients, chiropractors use methods that are specifically tailored to their needs. Children's bodies are still developing, so adjustments must be gentle and safe. For infants, chiropractors use a technique called cranial-sacral therapy, which involves gentle pressure on the head and spine to help release any tension and promote relaxation. For older children, chiropractors may use manual adjustments or instrument-assisted techniques, such as the Activator Method or the Gonstead Technique, which use gentle force to adjust the spine.

Chiropractors also take into consideration the unique needs of children when creating a treatment plan. They may incorporate exercises, stretches, and lifestyle changes to help improve their overall health and well-being. For example, chiropractors may recommend specific exercises to help improve posture or strengthen the core muscles, which can help to prevent future injuries and promote better spinal health.

One of the benefits of chiropractic care for children is that it is a non-invasive and drug-free approach to healthcare. This can be especially important for parents who are hesitant to give their children medication or expose them to unnecessary medical procedures. Chiropractic care can help to address a variety of health issues in a safe and natural way.

However, it is important to note that chiropractic care is not appropriate for every child. Chiropractors will typically conduct a thorough exam and take a detailed medical history before recommending treatment. They will also work closely with the child's pediatrician or other healthcare provider to ensure that the child receives the best possible care.

In addition to addressing specific health concerns, chiropractic care can also help to promote better overall health and well-being for children. Regular adjustments can help to improve sleep quality, boost the immune system, and promote better digestion. Chiropractors can also provide guidance on proper nutrition and lifestyle habits that can help to support a child's health and development.

Common pediatric conditions treated

Chiropractic care is a holistic approach to healthcare that involves the manipulation of the spine and other joints to promote proper alignment and restore proper function to the nervous system. While many people associate chiropractic care with adults, it is also a safe and effective treatment option for children. In fact, many common pediatric conditions can be treated through chiropractic care.

One of the most common reasons parents bring their children to a chiropractor is to treat ear infections. Ear infections are a painful condition that can cause fever, ear pain, and difficulty sleeping. Chiropractic care can help by reducing inflammation and restoring proper drainage to the ears. This is achieved through gentle adjustments of the upper cervical spine and other areas of the body that can impact the function of the ears.

Another common condition treated through chiropractic care is colic. Colic is a condition that affects infants and is characterized by excessive crying and irritability. Chiropractic care can help by reducing tension in the baby's spine, allowing for better digestion and a reduction in the symptoms of colic.

Chiropractic care is also effective in treating asthma. Asthma is a chronic respiratory condition that causes difficulty breathing, coughing, and wheezing. Chiropractic care can help by reducing inflammation in the respiratory system and restoring proper function to the lungs. This is achieved through adjustments of the spine and other areas of the body that can impact the respiratory system.

Chiropractic care is also effective in treating ADHD. ADHD is a neurological condition that affects attention, behavior, and cognitive function. Chiropractic care can help by reducing tension in the spine and restoring proper function to the nervous system. This is achieved through adjustments of the spine and other areas of the body that can impact the nervous system.

Another common condition treated through chiropractic care is scoliosis. Scoliosis is a condition that affects the curvature of the spine. Chiropractic care can help by reducing tension in the muscles and restoring proper alignment to the spine. This is achieved through adjustments of the spine and other areas of the body that can impact the curvature of the spine.

Chiropractic care is also effective in treating sports injuries in children. Sports injuries are common in children who participate in sports and can cause pain, swelling, and limited mobility. Chiropractic care can help by reducing inflammation and restoring proper function to the affected area. This is achieved through adjustments of the spine and other areas of the body that can impact the function of the affected area.

In addition to treating specific conditions, chiropractic care can also help promote overall health and wellness in children. Regular adjustments can help improve immune function, promote better sleep, and improve mood and behavior.

When it comes to treating children, chiropractors use a gentle approach that is appropriate for the child's age and size. Adjustments may involve gentle pressure, stretches, and massage techniques that are designed to be safe and effective for children of all ages.

Chapter Seven

Chiropractic Care During Pregnancy

Chiropractic care during pregnancy is a natural and safe option for women who wish to maintain optimal health and wellness during their pregnancy. Many expectant mothers experience discomfort and pain during pregnancy, including back pain, headaches, and sciatica. Chiropractic care can help alleviate these symptoms, as well as improve overall health and well-being for both mother and baby.

Chiropractic care is a non-invasive approach to healthcare that focuses on the relationship between the spine and the nervous system. Chiropractors are trained to identify and correct misalignments in the spine, also known as subluxations, which can interfere with the proper function of the nervous system. By restoring proper alignment and function to the spine, chiropractic care can improve overall health and wellness.

During pregnancy, the body undergoes many changes that can lead to subluxations in the spine. As the baby grows, the mother's center of gravity shifts forward, putting additional strain on the spine and pelvis. Hormonal changes also loosen ligaments and joints, which can contribute to misalignments in the spine. These subluxations can lead to pain and discomfort for the mother, as well as interfere with the proper development of the baby.

Chiropractic care can help address these issues and improve overall health and wellness during pregnancy. Chiropractors are trained to use techniques that are safe and effective for pregnant women, such as the Webster Technique. The Webster Technique is a specific chiropractic technique that focuses on the alignment of the pelvis, and is commonly used to address issues such as breech presentation.

In addition to addressing specific issues, chiropractic care can also help promote overall health and well-being during pregnancy. Regular adjustments can help improve the immune system, reduce stress and anxiety, and improve sleep quality. These benefits can help improve the mother's health and wellness, as well as promote healthy development for the baby.

Chiropractic care during pregnancy is generally considered safe, as long as the chiropractor is properly trained and experienced in working with pregnant women. Chiropractors may modify their techniques to accommodate the changing needs of the pregnant body, and may use special pillows or tables to ensure comfort and safety during adjustments.

It is important to note that while chiropractic care can be a valuable tool during pregnancy, it is not a substitute for traditional prenatal care. Women should continue to see their obstetrician or midwife for regular check-ups and screenings, as well as follow a healthy diet and exercise regimen.

Benefits and safety

Chiropractic care during pregnancy has gained popularity over the years as a safe and effective way to support the health and well-being of expectant mothers. As pregnancy progresses, the body undergoes a multitude of changes to accommodate the growing fetus, which can lead to discomfort and pain. Chiropractic adjustments can help alleviate these symptoms and promote overall health for both the mother and the baby.

One of the main benefits of chiropractic care during pregnancy is the reduction of lower back pain, which is a common complaint among expectant mothers. As the fetus grows, the center of gravity shifts, and the pelvis begins to tilt forward. This can lead to an increased curve in the lower back, which can cause muscle tension and pain. Chiropractic adjustments can help realign the spine and pelvis, reducing pressure on the lower back and relieving pain.

Chiropractic care can also improve overall spinal health during pregnancy. The hormonal changes that occur during pregnancy can cause ligaments to become lax, which can affect the stability of the spine. Chiropractic adjustments can help maintain spinal alignment and prevent the development of spinal problems.

Another benefit of chiropractic care during pregnancy is improved nervous system function. As the uterus expands, it can put pressure on the nerves that run through the pelvis and down the legs, leading to pain and discomfort. Chiropractic adjustments can help alleviate this pressure, improving nervous system function and reducing pain.

Chiropractic care is generally considered safe during pregnancy, as long as it is performed by a licensed chiropractor who is experienced in treating pregnant women. Pregnant women should inform their chiropractor about their pregnancy and any related health concerns. Chiropractors may use special techniques or equipment, such as pregnancy pillows or tables that can accommodate a growing belly, to ensure the comfort and safety of the mother and the baby.

It is important to note that certain conditions may make chiropractic care during pregnancy not advisable. Pregnant women with placenta previa, vaginal bleeding, or a history of preterm labor should consult with their healthcare provider before seeking chiropractic care. In addition, some chiropractic techniques, such as high-velocity adjustments, may not be appropriate during pregnancy.

Adjusting techniques for pregnant patients

Chiropractic care is a natural and non-invasive approach to health care that focuses on the spine and nervous system. It has been shown to be safe and effective for people of all ages, including pregnant women. Many pregnant women experience discomfort or pain during pregnancy due to the changes in their bodies, and chiropractic care can help alleviate these symptoms.

Chiropractic care during pregnancy can help prepare the body for labor and delivery, as well as promote the health of both the mother and baby. It can also help reduce the need for pain medication during delivery, as well as reduce the likelihood of interventions such as cesarean section.

However, when it comes to adjusting techniques for pregnant patients, chiropractors need to be particularly careful and use appropriate techniques to ensure the safety of both the mother and baby. Below we will explore some of the adjusting techniques used for pregnant patients.

The first technique used for pregnant patients is called the Webster Technique. This technique is specifically designed for pregnant women and involves adjusting the sacrum, or the triangular bone at the base of the spine. The goal of this technique is to improve the alignment of the pelvis, which can help reduce the likelihood of breech presentation and facilitate an easier delivery.

The Webster Technique involves a combination of adjustments, stretches, and soft tissue work. The chiropractor will begin by assessing the position of the pelvis and sacrum. If misalignments are found, the chiropractor will use gentle adjustments to realign the pelvis and reduce tension in the surrounding muscles and ligaments.

Another adjusting technique used for pregnant patients is the Logan Basic Technique. This technique involves applying gentle pressure to the sacrum using a specialized table. The goal of this technique is to reduce tension in the muscles and ligaments surrounding the sacrum, which can help improve the alignment of the pelvis.

The Logan Basic Technique is gentle and safe for pregnant patients, and can help alleviate low back pain and other discomforts associated with pregnancy.

The third technique used for pregnant patients is called the Activator Method. This technique involves the use of a small hand-held instrument that delivers a precise and gentle force to the spine. The Activator Method is particularly useful for pregnant patients, as it does not involve any twisting or bending of the spine.

The Activator Method is safe and effective for pregnant patients, and can help reduce pain and discomfort associated with pregnancy. It can also help improve the alignment of the spine and reduce tension in the muscles and ligaments.

Chiropractors also use soft tissue techniques to help pregnant patients. These techniques involve the use of massage, stretching, and other manual techniques to reduce tension in the muscles and improve circulation. Soft tissue techniques can help reduce pain and discomfort associated with pregnancy, as well as promote relaxation and stress reduction.

In addition to these adjusting techniques, chiropractors may also recommend exercises and stretches that can be done at home to help promote spinal health during pregnancy. These exercises are gentle and safe for pregnant patients, and can help reduce tension in the muscles and improve circulation.

Alleviating pregnancy-related discomfort

Chiropractic care can be beneficial for pregnant women who experience discomfort or pain during their pregnancy. Many women experience back pain, hip pain, and other musculoskeletal issues during pregnancy due to changes in weight distribution and hormonal changes. Chiropractic care can provide a safe and effective way to alleviate these symptoms.

Chiropractors use a variety of adjusting techniques that are safe for pregnant women. The techniques used will depend on the individual needs of the patient and may include low-force techniques such as the activator method or gentle spinal mobilization. Chiropractors may also use special pillows and tables to accommodate the growing belly and ensure the safety and comfort of the patient.

One of the most common conditions that chiropractors treat during pregnancy is low back pain. As the baby grows, the center of gravity shifts forward, which can cause strain on the lower back muscles and ligaments. Chiropractors can use spinal adjustments and soft tissue techniques to relieve tension and improve mobility in the lower back. In addition to chiropractic care, pregnant women may also benefit from exercises that strengthen the lower back and pelvic muscles.

Chiropractic care may also be beneficial for pregnant women experiencing sciatica, which is pain that radiates from the lower back down to the legs. Sciatica can be caused by pressure on the sciatic nerve, which can occur during pregnancy due to the weight of the baby. Chiropractic adjustments can help alleviate the pressure on the nerve and relieve the pain.

Another common condition that pregnant women may experience is pubic symphysis dysfunction, which is pain and inflammation in the pubic area. This condition occurs when the hormone relaxin, which is released during pregnancy, causes the ligaments in the pelvis to become more relaxed, resulting in instability in the pubic area. Chiropractors can use gentle mobilization techniques and exercises to alleviate this pain and restore stability to the pelvis.

In addition to alleviating musculoskeletal pain and discomfort, chiropractic care may also provide other benefits for pregnant women. Studies have shown that chiropractic care can reduce the length of labor and decrease the need for medical interventions during delivery. Chiropractic care can also help improve sleep quality, reduce stress and anxiety, and improve overall well-being during pregnancy.

It is important to note that pregnant women should always consult with their healthcare provider before seeking chiropractic care. Chiropractors who specialize in prenatal care will also take precautions to ensure the safety of the mother and baby. For example, chiropractors will avoid certain techniques and areas of the body that may be contraindicated during pregnancy.

Chapter Eight

Preventative Care and Maintenance

Preventive care and maintenance are essential aspects of overall health and wellness. Chiropractic care can be an important part of preventative care and maintenance, helping to keep the body in proper alignment and function optimally. Below we will explore the benefits of chiropractic care as a preventative measure, as well as the techniques and strategies used to maintain health and wellness.

One of the primary benefits of chiropractic care is its focus on maintaining the proper alignment of the spine. The spine is the body's central support structure, and it houses the nervous system that controls all of the body's functions. When the spine is misaligned, it can lead to a wide range of health problems, including pain, reduced mobility, and decreased overall health and wellness.

Chiropractic care seeks to maintain proper spinal alignment by using a range of techniques, including spinal manipulation, mobilization, and soft tissue techniques. These techniques are designed to help restore proper alignment and range of motion in the spine, allowing the body to function at its best.

In addition to maintaining proper spinal alignment, chiropractic care can also help prevent injuries and illnesses. By addressing issues with the spine and nervous system, chiropractors can help identify potential problem areas and work to correct them before they become more serious. This proactive approach to healthcare can help patients avoid more invasive and costly treatments down the road.

Another benefit of chiropractic care as a preventative measure is that it is non-invasive and drug-free. Chiropractors focus on using natural, holistic methods to help the body heal and maintain its health. This approach can be particularly beneficial for individuals who are looking to avoid the potential side effects of medications or who are seeking a more natural approach to healthcare.

Chiropractic care can also be customized to meet the unique needs of each patient. Chiropractors work closely with their patients to develop personalized treatment plans that take into account their health history, lifestyle, and overall health goals. By tailoring their approach to each individual patient, chiropractors can provide more effective and targeted care.

One important aspect of preventative care and maintenance in chiropractic is the concept of wellness care. Wellness care is a proactive approach to healthcare that focuses on maintaining optimal health and wellness through regular checkups, adjustments, and other preventative measures. By engaging in wellness care, patients can stay ahead of potential health problems and maintain their overall health and well-being.

To maintain optimal health and wellness through chiropractic care, patients may undergo regular spinal adjustments, nutritional counseling, and lifestyle coaching. These services are designed to help patients maintain proper spinal alignment, improve their diet and exercise habits, and reduce stress levels. By addressing these key areas of health and wellness, patients can experience improved overall health and a reduced risk of illness and injury.

In addition to spinal adjustments and lifestyle counseling, chiropractors may also recommend other preventative measures, such as massage therapy, acupuncture, and other complementary therapies. These treatments can help promote relaxation, reduce stress levels, and improve overall health and well-being.

Posture and ergonomics

Posture and ergonomics are important factors that can have a significant impact on our health and well-being. Poor posture and ergonomic habits can lead to a range of issues such as back pain, headaches, and joint problems. Chiropractors play an important role in educating patients about posture and ergonomics, and providing treatments to help improve posture and prevent related health problems.

Posture refers to the way we hold our body when sitting, standing, or moving. Good posture means that our body is in proper alignment, with our weight evenly distributed throughout our spine and limbs. Poor posture, on the other hand, means that our body is out of alignment, putting extra strain on certain muscles and joints. This can lead to a range of issues, including back pain, neck pain, and headaches.

Ergonomics, on the other hand, refers to the design of our work and living environments, and how these designs affect our posture and overall health. For example, an office chair that is not properly adjusted can lead to poor posture and back pain, while a poorly designed computer monitor can cause eye strain and headaches.

Chiropractors are trained to assess posture and ergonomic habits, and can provide patients with recommendations on how to improve both. This may include advice on how to sit and stand properly, how to adjust office chairs and computer monitors, and how to improve overall body mechanics during daily activities. Chiropractors may also provide hands-on treatments, such as spinal adjustments, soft tissue therapy, and exercises, to help patients improve their posture and prevent related health problems.

One of the most common issues related to poor posture is back pain. Back pain affects millions of people worldwide, and is one of the leading causes of disability. Poor posture, such as slouching or hunching over, can put extra strain on the muscles and ligaments of the back, leading to pain and discomfort. Chiropractors can help alleviate back pain by identifying and treating the underlying causes, including poor posture and ergonomic habits. This may involve spinal adjustments, soft tissue therapy, and exercises to improve spinal alignment and muscle strength.

Another common issue related to poor posture is neck pain. Neck pain is often caused by poor posture habits, such as hunching over a computer or phone screen for extended periods of time. Chiropractors can help alleviate neck pain by identifying and treating the underlying causes, including poor posture and ergonomic habits. This may involve spinal adjustments, soft tissue therapy, and exercises to improve spinal alignment and muscle strength.

Headaches are also a common issue related to poor posture and ergonomics. Poor posture can lead to tension headaches, while poor ergonomics, such as improperly positioned computer monitors, can lead to eyestrain and headaches. Chiropractors can help alleviate headaches by identifying and treating the underlying causes, including poor posture and ergonomic habits. This may involve spinal adjustments, soft tissue therapy, and exercises to improve spinal alignment and muscle strength.

In addition to treating existing health problems related to poor posture and ergonomics, chiropractors can also help prevent future health problems. By providing education and hands-on treatments, chiropractors can help patients develop good posture habits and ergonomic practices that can prevent health problems from developing in the first place.

Exercise and stretching

Chiropractic care is not only about adjustments and spinal manipulation; it also involves educating patients about lifestyle habits and practices that can support their overall health and well-being. Exercise and stretching are two crucial aspects of this preventative care and maintenance approach.

Exercise is vital for maintaining flexibility, strength, and range of motion. Regular physical activity can improve joint function and reduce the risk of injury. Chiropractors often recommend exercises that target specific muscle groups and promote proper alignment and posture. The exercises prescribed may depend on the patient's age, physical condition, and health goals.

For example, a chiropractor may recommend exercises to help improve core strength, which can help support the spine and reduce the risk of back pain. Strengthening exercises for the back muscles can also help alleviate tension and tightness in the spine. Patients may also receive guidance on exercises that can be done to support specific conditions such as neck pain or sciatica.

In addition to exercise, stretching is also an essential component of chiropractic care. Stretching can help improve flexibility and range of motion and reduce muscle tension. Chiropractors may recommend specific stretching techniques to alleviate tightness in particular areas of the body. For instance, stretching the hamstrings can help reduce lower back pain by improving pelvic alignment.

Chiropractors may also teach patients stretching techniques to use at home. These techniques may be tailored to address the patient's specific condition and may include stretching the neck, shoulders, hips, and legs. Patients may also be instructed on how to use foam rollers or other tools to perform self-myofascial release, which can help release muscle tension and improve mobility.

Chiropractors may also recommend other forms of exercise, such as yoga or Pilates, which can help improve posture and balance, strengthen core muscles, and increase flexibility. These forms of exercise can also promote relaxation and reduce stress, which can have a positive impact on overall health.

It's important to note that patients should consult with their chiropractor before beginning any exercise or stretching program. Chiropractors can provide guidance on the best exercises and techniques for each patient's specific needs and goals. Patients should also inform their chiropractor of any pain or discomfort they experience during exercise or stretching.

Chiropractors may also recommend modifications to the patient's daily routine to support spinal health. For example, they may provide guidance on proper ergonomics for desk work or recommend adjustments to the patient's sleeping position. These modifications can help reduce stress on the spine and improve posture, reducing the risk of injury or discomfort.

Nutrition and supplements

Chiropractic care is a holistic approach to healthcare that focuses on the relationship between the spine and the nervous system. While many people associate chiropractic care with spinal adjustments, there are many other aspects to this form of treatment that can promote overall health and well-being. One of these aspects is nutrition and supplements.

Nutrition and supplements play a crucial role in overall health and wellness. Proper nutrition can help reduce inflammation, promote healing, and support a healthy immune system. Supplements can provide additional support for the body in the form of vitamins, minerals, and other nutrients that may be lacking in a person's diet. Chiropractors recognize the importance of nutrition and supplements in promoting optimal health and may incorporate these into their treatment plans.

Chiropractors can provide guidance on proper nutrition and may recommend supplements to address specific health concerns. For example, if a person is experiencing joint pain or inflammation, the chiropractor may recommend supplements such as omega-3 fatty acids or turmeric, which have been shown to have anti-inflammatory effects. They may also recommend supplements to support bone health, such as vitamin D and calcium.

In addition to recommending supplements, chiropractors may also provide guidance on healthy eating habits. This can include advice on portion control, balanced meals, and avoiding processed foods. Chiropractors can also provide guidance on dietary changes that may be beneficial for specific health concerns, such as reducing sugar intake to improve blood sugar control in people with diabetes.

Chiropractors may also incorporate nutritional counseling into their treatment plans. This involves reviewing a person's current diet and making recommendations for improvements. Nutritional counseling may also involve providing education on the benefits of certain foods and how to incorporate them into a person's diet.

It is important to note that while chiropractors can provide guidance on nutrition and supplements, they are not licensed to provide medical nutrition therapy. This is a specialized field that involves diagnosing and treating specific medical conditions through nutrition interventions. If a person has a specific medical condition that requires medical nutrition therapy, they should consult a registered dietitian or other qualified healthcare provider.

In addition to providing guidance on nutrition and supplements, chiropractors may also incorporate lifestyle modifications into their treatment plans. This can include recommendations for exercise and stretching to improve mobility and flexibility. Chiropractors can also provide guidance on proper posture and ergonomics to prevent injury and improve overall spinal health.

Chapter Nine

Chiropractic and Integrative Healthcare

Chiropractic is a form of healthcare that focuses on the diagnosis and treatment of neuromuscular disorders, with an emphasis on the spine and its impact on overall health. Chiropractors use manual therapies, including spinal manipulation, to improve joint function, reduce pain, and restore range of motion. While chiropractic is often considered a standalone form of healthcare, it can also be integrated with other forms of complementary and alternative medicine to provide a more comprehensive approach to patient care.

Integrative healthcare is an approach that combines conventional medicine with complementary and alternative therapies to promote healing and wellness. Chiropractic is one of the many forms of complementary and alternative medicine that can be integrated into a patient's overall healthcare plan. Integrative healthcare is based on the idea that every person is unique, and that there is no one-size-fits-all approach to health and wellness. Instead, integrative healthcare takes a holistic approach to patient care, focusing on the physical, emotional, and spiritual aspects of health and wellness.

Chiropractic care can be integrated with a wide range of other therapies, including massage therapy, acupuncture, nutritional counseling, and herbal medicine. By combining different forms of therapy, chiropractors can provide a more comprehensive approach to patient care that addresses the root cause of health problems rather than just treating symptoms.

One of the key benefits of integrative healthcare is that it can help patients achieve better outcomes than traditional medicine alone. By combining different forms of therapy, integrative healthcare can help patients manage their symptoms more effectively, reduce the risk of side effects, and improve their overall quality of life.

For example, chiropractic care can be used to treat a wide range of musculoskeletal problems, including back pain, neck pain, and headaches. Massage therapy can be used to reduce muscle tension and improve circulation, while acupuncture can be used to reduce pain and promote healing. Nutritional counseling and herbal medicine can be used to address nutritional deficiencies and support the body's natural healing processes.

Integrative healthcare can also be used to treat chronic conditions such as diabetes, high blood pressure, and cardiovascular disease. By combining different forms of therapy, integrative healthcare can help patients manage these conditions more effectively and reduce the risk of complications.

In addition to its effectiveness, integrative healthcare is also safe and natural. Unlike conventional medicine, which often relies on drugs and surgery to treat health problems, integrative healthcare focuses on natural therapies that work with the body's natural healing processes. This means that integrative healthcare is often less invasive, less risky, and less costly than traditional medicine.

One of the challenges of integrative healthcare is that it can be difficult to find healthcare providers who are trained in both conventional medicine and complementary and alternative medicine. However, as integrative healthcare becomes more popular, more healthcare providers are becoming trained in these different forms of therapy, making it easier for patients to find the care they need.

Combining chiropractic with other therapies

Chiropractic care has been used to treat a wide range of conditions, from back pain and headaches to sports injuries and pregnancy-related discomfort. While chiropractic is often seen as a standalone therapy, it can also be combined with other treatments to create an integrated approach to healthcare. Below we will we'll explore the benefits of combining chiropractic with other therapies and some of the most popular treatment options.

Integrative healthcare is becoming more popular, and it's easy to see why. When different therapies are combined, they can often work together to achieve better results than each therapy could on its own. Chiropractic care is a perfect example of a therapy that can be combined with others to create an integrated approach to healthcare. By treating the spine and nervous system, chiropractic can improve overall health and well-being. When combined with other therapies, such as massage or acupuncture, the results can be even more impressive.

One of the most popular therapies to combine with chiropractic care is massage therapy. Massage and chiropractic work together to address musculoskeletal problems and promote relaxation. Massage can help to relax the muscles, making it easier for the chiropractor to adjust the spine. Chiropractic adjustments can then help to improve circulation and nerve function, enhancing the benefits of the massage.

Another therapy commonly combined with chiropractic is acupuncture. Acupuncture is a traditional Chinese therapy that involves inserting thin needles into specific points on the body to promote healing. Acupuncture can be used to relieve pain and improve overall health, and it works particularly well when combined with chiropractic. Chiropractic adjustments can help to relieve muscle tension and improve spinal alignment, while acupuncture can address issues like inflammation and stress.

In addition to massage and acupuncture, there are many other therapies that can be combined with chiropractic care. For example, yoga and Pilates can help to improve flexibility and core strength, which can enhance the results of chiropractic adjustments. Nutritional counseling can also be helpful, as proper nutrition can help to support overall health and well-being.

When combining chiropractic with other therapies, it's important to work with healthcare professionals who are experienced in integrative healthcare. This will ensure that the different therapies are used in a safe and effective way. Patients should also be sure to discuss any existing health conditions or concerns with their chiropractor and other healthcare providers.

Integrative healthcare has many benefits, and combining chiropractic with other therapies can lead to better results than each therapy could achieve on its own. By addressing the whole person and using a variety of therapies, integrative healthcare can help to promote overall health and well-being. Whether you're dealing with back pain, headaches, or other health issues, combining chiropractic care with other therapies can be a great way to improve your health and feel your best.

Multidisciplinary care approach

Multidisciplinary care is a healthcare approach that involves professionals from multiple disciplines working collaboratively to provide comprehensive care to patients. In recent years, this approach has gained increasing popularity in the field of chiropractic care as a way to provide patients with more holistic, integrated care.

Chiropractic care is a non-invasive, drug-free approach to healthcare that focuses on the diagnosis, treatment, and prevention of musculoskeletal disorders, particularly those related to the spine. Chiropractors use a variety of techniques, including spinal manipulation, mobilization, soft tissue therapy, and exercise and stretching, to improve the function of the nervous and musculoskeletal systems and alleviate pain and discomfort.

While chiropractic care can be effective on its own, combining it with other therapies can enhance its benefits and lead to better outcomes for patients. Multidisciplinary care approaches may involve working with other healthcare professionals, such as physical therapists, massage therapists, acupuncturists, and nutritionists, to provide patients with a more comprehensive approach to care.

One of the primary benefits of a multidisciplinary care approach is the ability to address the root causes of a patient's condition from multiple angles. For example, if a patient is experiencing back pain, a chiropractor may provide spinal manipulation and mobilization to realign the spine and reduce tension in the surrounding muscles. However, if the pain is due to poor posture, a physical therapist may work with the patient to develop a stretching and exercise program to strengthen the muscles and improve alignment. Additionally, a nutritionist may work with the patient to develop a healthy eating plan to reduce inflammation and improve overall health.

By working collaboratively with other healthcare professionals, chiropractors can provide patients with a more integrated approach to care, addressing all aspects of their health and well-being. This approach can lead to better outcomes and improved quality of life for patients.

Another benefit of multidisciplinary care is the ability to tailor treatment plans to individual patient needs. Every patient is unique, with their own set of health concerns and goals for treatment. By working with a team of healthcare professionals, chiropractors can develop individualized treatment plans that take into account each patient's specific needs and preferences.

For example, if a patient is uncomfortable with spinal manipulation, a chiropractor may work with a massage therapist to provide soft tissue therapy and mobilization techniques instead. By taking into account the patient's comfort level and preferences, the multidisciplinary care team can provide a more customized approach to care that meets the needs of each individual patient.

In addition to improving outcomes and providing individualized care, multidisciplinary care can also help reduce healthcare costs. By addressing all aspects of a patient's health and well-being, including nutrition, exercise, and stress management, multidisciplinary care can help prevent the need for costly interventions such as surgery or long-term medication use.

Furthermore, by working collaboratively with other healthcare professionals, chiropractors can refer patients to other specialists as needed, preventing unnecessary testing and procedures and reducing overall healthcare costs.

Chiropractic in the healthcare system

Chiropractic is a healthcare profession that focuses on diagnosing, treating, and preventing musculoskeletal disorders and their effects on the nervous system and general health. Although it is considered an alternative therapy, chiropractic is becoming more integrated into the mainstream healthcare system due to its effectiveness in treating a wide range of conditions.

Chiropractic is founded on the principles that the body has an innate ability to heal itself and that proper alignment of the musculoskeletal system is essential to overall health and wellbeing. Chiropractors use non-invasive, drug-free techniques to restore proper alignment and function of the spine and other joints, which can relieve pain, improve mobility, and enhance overall health.

Chiropractic care can be used as a standalone therapy or in combination with other treatments. The most common conditions treated by chiropractors include back pain, neck pain, headaches, and sports injuries. However, chiropractic has been shown to be effective in treating a wide range of conditions, including asthma, allergies, digestive disorders, and even ADHD.

One of the benefits of chiropractic care is its ability to complement other healthcare practices. Chiropractors often work alongside medical doctors, physical therapists, and other healthcare professionals to provide a multidisciplinary approach to patient care. This approach allows for a more comprehensive assessment of the patient's condition and provides more opportunities for collaboration and improved patient outcomes.

Chiropractors often use a combination of techniques in their practice, including spinal manipulation, mobilization, and soft tissue therapy. Spinal manipulation is a technique that involves applying a controlled force to a joint in the spine to restore its normal motion and alignment. Mobilization is a gentler technique that involves moving a joint through its natural range of motion to improve mobility and reduce pain. Soft tissue therapy involves applying pressure to muscles and other soft tissues to relieve tension and improve circulation.

Chiropractors also focus on preventative care and maintenance, including education on posture and ergonomics, exercise and stretching, and nutrition and supplements. By promoting healthy habits and lifestyle choices, chiropractors can help their patients maintain optimal musculoskeletal and nervous system health and prevent future problems.

The integration of chiropractic into the healthcare system has been increasing in recent years. Many hospitals and medical clinics now have chiropractors on staff or work closely with chiropractic clinics to provide comprehensive patient care. Insurance companies are also recognizing the benefits of chiropractic care and are beginning to cover it as a standard healthcare practice.

Chapter Ten

Choosing a Chiropractor

Choosing a chiropractor can be a daunting task, especially if you have never visited one before. Chiropractic care is a specialized field, and it's important to choose a chiropractor who is experienced, knowledgeable, and trustworthy. Below we will discuss some of the key factors to consider when choosing a chiropractor.

First and foremost, it's important to ensure that the chiropractor you choose is licensed and registered. In the United States, chiropractors are licensed by state regulatory boards. You can verify a chiropractor's license by contacting your state's chiropractic board. Additionally, it's important to check whether the chiropractor has any malpractice claims or disciplinary actions on their record. This information can be found on the state's licensing website or the National Practitioner Data Bank.

Once you have verified the chiropractor's credentials, it's important to consider their experience and expertise. You may want to ask the chiropractor about their education, training, and areas of specialization. Chiropractors may have expertise in treating specific conditions such as sports injuries, back pain, or neck pain. It's important to choose a chiropractor whose expertise aligns with your specific needs.

Another factor to consider when choosing a chiropractor is their communication style. The chiropractor should be able to explain their diagnosis and treatment plan in a way that you can understand. They should also be willing to answer any questions you may have and address any concerns you may have about the treatment. It's important to choose a chiropractor who listens to your concerns and takes the time to understand your needs.

In addition to the chiropractor's communication style, you may also want to consider their treatment approach. Chiropractors may use a variety of techniques such as spinal manipulation, mobilization, soft tissue techniques, and rehabilitation exercises. It's important to choose a chiropractor whose treatment approach aligns with your personal preferences and comfort level. For example, if you prefer gentle manipulation techniques, you may want to choose a chiropractor who specializes in these techniques.

Another important factor to consider when choosing a chiropractor is their availability and location. You may want to choose a chiropractor who is located close to your home or workplace for convenience. Additionally, you may want to consider their availability for appointments, especially if you have a busy schedule.

Lastly, it's important to consider the chiropractor's fees and insurance coverage. Chiropractic care may not be covered by all insurance plans, so it's important to check your coverage before scheduling an appointment. You may also want to inquire about the chiropractor's fees for treatment and any additional services they offer such as x-rays or other diagnostic tests.

Licensing and credentials

Chiropractic is a type of complementary medicine that focuses on the musculoskeletal system, particularly the spine, with the goal of improving overall health and well-being. To become a licensed chiropractor, individuals must complete an extensive educational program and meet specific requirements for licensing and credentialing. Below we will explore the licensing and credentialing requirements for chiropractors, the importance of selecting a licensed chiropractor, and the benefits of seeking chiropractic care from a licensed and credentialed professional.

In the United States, chiropractors are licensed by each state and the District of Columbia. The requirements for licensure vary from state to state, but generally include completion of a Doctor of Chiropractic (DC) program from an accredited college of chiropractic, passing the National Board of Chiropractic Examiners (NBCE) exams, and completing a certain number of hours of supervised clinical experience.

The DC program typically takes four years to complete and includes coursework in anatomy, physiology, pathology, biomechanics, and chiropractic techniques. Students also gain hands-on experience in diagnosing and treating patients under the supervision of licensed chiropractors.

After completing the DC program, individuals must pass the NBCE exams, which include written and practical sections. The exams assess knowledge and skills related to chiropractic diagnosis, treatment, and patient care.

In addition to completing the DC program and passing the NBCE exams, individuals must also complete a certain number of hours of supervised clinical experience to be eligible for licensure. These requirements vary by state, but typically range from 500 to 1,000 hours.

Once licensed, chiropractors must maintain their credentials by completing continuing education courses to stay up-to-date on the latest developments in chiropractic care. Continuing education requirements vary by state but generally require chiropractors to complete a certain number of hours of coursework every year or every two years.

It is important for patients to choose a licensed and credentialed chiropractor to ensure that they receive safe and effective care. Licensed chiropractors have completed the necessary education and training to diagnose and treat musculoskeletal conditions and have passed rigorous exams to demonstrate their competency in the field.

Patients should also look for chiropractors who are members of professional organizations, such as the American Chiropractic Association or the International Chiropractors Association, which require members to adhere to high standards of ethics and professionalism.

Choosing a licensed and credentialed chiropractor can also help patients avoid the potential risks associated with unlicensed and untrained individuals who may offer chiropractic services. These risks can include misdiagnosis, inappropriate treatment, and exacerbation of existing conditions.

In addition to providing safe and effective care, seeking chiropractic treatment from a licensed and credentialed professional can offer numerous benefits for patients. Chiropractic care has been shown to be effective in treating a variety of musculoskeletal conditions, including back pain, neck pain, and headaches. It can also help improve joint mobility, reduce inflammation, and enhance overall physical performance.

Chiropractors can also work in conjunction with other healthcare professionals, such as physical therapists and primary care physicians, to provide a comprehensive approach to patient care. This multidisciplinary approach can help ensure that patients receive the most appropriate and effective treatment for their specific condition.

Finding the right practitioner

Finding the right chiropractor can be a daunting task, especially if you are new to chiropractic care. However, with a few simple steps, you can find a qualified practitioner who can help you achieve your health goals. Below we will discuss some tips for finding the right chiropractor.

The first step in finding the right chiropractor is to ask for recommendations. You can ask your friends, family, or colleagues if they know of any good chiropractors in your area. If you know someone who has received chiropractic care, they can give you valuable insights into the chiropractor's quality of care, bedside manner, and overall experience.

Once you have a list of potential chiropractors, it's important to research each one thoroughly. You can start by checking their credentials and licensing. Make sure that the chiropractor is licensed to practice in your state and has completed the required education and training. You can also check if the chiropractor has any disciplinary actions or malpractice claims against them.

Next, take a look at the chiropractor's experience and expertise. Some chiropractors specialize in certain areas such as sports injuries or pediatric care. If you have a specific health concern, it's important to find a chiropractor who has experience in treating that condition. You can check the chiropractor's website or call their office to find out more about their expertise.

Another important factor to consider is the chiropractor's approach to treatment. Some chiropractors focus solely on spinal manipulation, while others incorporate other techniques such as massage therapy or acupuncture. It's important to find a chiropractor whose approach aligns with your health goals and preferences.

When you have narrowed down your list of potential chiropractors, it's a good idea to schedule a consultation or initial appointment. This will give you the opportunity to meet the chiropractor in person, discuss your health concerns, and ask any questions you may have. Pay attention to how the chiropractor communicates with you and whether they listen to your concerns.

During your appointment, the chiropractor may also perform a physical exam or order diagnostic tests such as x-rays or MRI scans. This can help them determine the cause of your symptoms and develop an appropriate treatment plan. If you feel uncomfortable or uneasy during the exam or tests, it's important to speak up and let the chiropractor know.

Finally, consider the cost and insurance coverage. Chiropractic care can be expensive, and it's important to find a chiropractor who accepts your insurance or offers affordable payment options. You can also check if the chiropractor offers a free initial consultation or package deals for multiple visits.

Questions to ask during your first visit

Chiropractic care is a popular form of complementary and alternative medicine that focuses on the diagnosis, treatment, and prevention of mechanical disorders of the musculoskeletal system, particularly the spine. If you're considering chiropractic care, it's essential to find the right practitioner and ask the right questions to ensure that you receive safe and effective care. Below we will we'll discuss some of the questions you should ask during your first visit with a chiropractor.

What is your educational background and credentials?

It's crucial to know the education and credentials of your chiropractor before receiving treatment. Chiropractors must complete a rigorous educational program, including a four-year chiropractic degree program and a supervised clinical internship. Look for chiropractors who have received their degrees from accredited institutions and who are licensed to practice in your state.

What is your treatment philosophy?

Every chiropractor has a unique approach to treatment. Some chiropractors may use a variety of techniques, while others may specialize in one particular method. It's important to find a chiropractor who aligns with your personal preferences and values.

Can you explain the treatment plan?

Before starting treatment, your chiropractor should provide a detailed treatment plan that outlines the recommended course of treatment, the expected timeline, and the estimated cost. A good chiropractor should be transparent about their approach and provide a clear and concise explanation of the treatment plan.

What are the potential risks and side effects?

Like any medical treatment, chiropractic care comes with potential risks and side effects. Before beginning treatment, your chiropractor should explain the possible risks and side effects associated with the specific techniques they use. They should also discuss any precautions you should take to avoid injury or discomfort during treatment.

Can you provide references or testimonials?

If you're considering a chiropractor, it's essential to ask for references or testimonials from previous patients. This will give you a better understanding of their experience with the chiropractor and the effectiveness of the treatment they received.

Do you accept insurance, and what are the payment options?

Chiropractic care can be costly, so it's important to know if your chiropractor accepts insurance and what payment options are available. Some chiropractors offer payment plans or may accept credit cards, while others may require full payment upfront.

How long will the treatment take, and how many visits will I need?

The duration of chiropractic treatment can vary depending on the nature and severity of your condition. Your chiropractor should be able to provide an estimate of how long treatment will take and how many visits you'll need. They should also be willing to adjust the treatment plan based on your progress and response to treatment.

What can I expect during treatment?

Before beginning treatment, your chiropractor should explain what to expect during treatment. This may include information on the specific techniques used, the duration of the treatment, and any potential sensations or discomfort you may experience.

Chapter Eleven

Your First Chiropractic Appointment

If you have never visited a chiropractor before, you may be unsure of what to expect during your first appointment. Below we will provide an overview of what typically happens during a first chiropractic appointment and what you can do to make the most of your experience.

The first step in your chiropractic journey is to find a chiropractor in your area. You can do this by asking for recommendations from friends and family, doing an online search, or checking with your insurance provider. Once you have found a chiropractor, you will need to schedule an appointment.

Before Your Appointment

When you call to schedule your appointment, the office staff will likely ask you to fill out some paperwork. This paperwork may include a health history form, a consent form, and a privacy policy. You can often find these forms on the chiropractor's website and complete them before your appointment to save time.

It's also a good idea to wear comfortable clothing to your appointment, as you may be asked to change into a gown or shorts for the exam. Avoid wearing anything that is tight or restricts movement.

During Your Appointment

When you arrive for your appointment, you will likely be greeted by the chiropractor or a member of the office staff. They may ask you to fill out any remaining paperwork or update your health history.

Next, the chiropractor will conduct a physical exam, which may include a range of motion tests, posture analysis, and palpation of the spine and surrounding muscles. They may also use diagnostic tools such as x-rays or MRI scans to help identify any underlying issues.

Based on the results of the exam, the chiropractor will develop a treatment plan that is tailored to your specific needs. This may include adjustments, soft tissue therapy, exercises, and lifestyle recommendations.

The adjustment itself is a gentle, non-invasive technique that involves applying controlled pressure to specific joints in the spine. The chiropractor will use their hands or a specialized tool to deliver the adjustment, which can help improve joint function, reduce pain, and improve overall mobility.

After Your Appointment

After your appointment, the chiropractor will likely provide you with some guidance on what to expect in the coming days and weeks. They may suggest specific exercises or stretches to help you maintain your progress between appointments.

It's important to follow any instructions provided by your chiropractor, as this can help you get the most out of your treatment. You may also be asked to schedule follow-up appointments to continue your care.

If you experience any pain or discomfort after your appointment, don't hesitate to reach out to your chiropractor for guidance. They can help you determine if this is a normal part of the healing process or if there is something more serious going on.

What to expect

Chiropractic is a type of healthcare that focuses on the diagnosis and treatment of musculoskeletal and nervous system disorders. It is a non-invasive and drug-free form of treatment that seeks to improve the body's natural ability to heal itself. If you're considering seeing a chiropractor for the first time, it's normal to feel a little nervous or unsure about what to expect. Below we will we'll explore what happens during a typical chiropractic appointment and what you can expect as a new patient.

Before the Appointment

Before your first chiropractic appointment, you'll typically need to fill out some paperwork. This paperwork will likely include a health history form, which will ask about any past injuries, surgeries, and medical conditions you've had. You may also need to sign a consent form, which will outline the risks and benefits of chiropractic care and your rights as a patient. Some chiropractic offices may also ask you to complete a pain questionnaire or a survey about your lifestyle habits.

The Initial Consultation

Your first chiropractic appointment will likely begin with an initial consultation. During this consultation, the chiropractor will ask you about your medical history, any current symptoms you're experiencing, and any activities that may be contributing to your pain. They may also ask about your lifestyle habits, such as your diet, exercise routine, and stress levels. The chiropractor will use this information to create a comprehensive picture of your overall health and any potential issues that may be contributing to your symptoms.

Physical Examination

After the initial consultation, the chiropractor will likely perform a physical examination. This examination may include a series of tests to evaluate your posture, balance, and range of motion. The chiropractor may also perform orthopedic and neurological tests to assess your joint function, muscle strength, and reflexes. Depending on your symptoms and medical history, the chiropractor may also perform additional tests such as X-rays or an MRI.

Chiropractic Adjustment

Once the chiropractor has completed their examination, they may perform a chiropractic adjustment. During this adjustment, the chiropractor will use their hands or a small tool to apply controlled force to specific joints in the spine. This force is designed to correct any misalignments, or subluxations, in the spine that may be causing pain or discomfort. Chiropractic adjustments are generally painless, although you may hear a popping or cracking sound as the joints are realigned.

Other Treatments

In addition to chiropractic adjustments, your chiropractor may also recommend other treatments to help alleviate your symptoms. These treatments may include:

1. Soft tissue therapy: This involves using massage or other techniques to loosen tight muscles and improve circulation.

2. Electrical stimulation: This involves using low-level electrical currents to stimulate the muscles and reduce pain.

3. Ice or heat therapy: This involves using ice or heat packs to reduce inflammation and promote healing.

4. Exercise and stretching: Your chiropractor may recommend specific exercises and stretches to help improve your flexibility and range of motion.

Follow-Up Appointments

After your initial appointment, your chiropractor will likely recommend a series of follow-up appointments. These appointments are designed to monitor your progress and make any necessary adjustments to your treatment plan. Depending on your symptoms and the severity of your condition, you may need to see your chiropractor once a week or once a month.

Patient consent and communication

Chiropractic care involves a lot of physical contact between the patient and the chiropractor. It is important for patients to have a clear understanding of what chiropractic care entails and to give informed consent before beginning any treatment. Effective communication between the patient and chiropractor is essential for ensuring that the patient is comfortable and informed throughout the treatment process. Below we will discuss the importance of patient consent and communication in chiropractic care.

Patient consent is a crucial component of chiropractic care. Patients have the right to make informed decisions about their health care, and this includes chiropractic treatment. Before beginning any treatment, the chiropractor should explain the treatment plan to the patient, including the potential risks and benefits. The patient should be given the opportunity to ask questions and express any concerns they may have. Once the patient fully understands the treatment plan, they can give their informed consent to proceed.

Chiropractors also need to be aware of any underlying health conditions that the patient may have. They should obtain a detailed medical history from the patient and perform a thorough examination to assess the patient's overall health. This is important because some health conditions may affect the type of treatment that can be used or may require modifications to the treatment plan.

Effective communication between the chiropractor and patient is crucial for the success of chiropractic care. Patients should feel comfortable discussing their symptoms, concerns, and expectations with their chiropractor. Likewise, chiropractors should be clear and concise when explaining treatment plans and answering questions. They should also provide patients with clear instructions on how to perform any exercises or stretches they may be given as part of their treatment plan.

In addition to verbal communication, nonverbal communication is also important in chiropractic care. Chiropractors should be aware of their body language and facial expressions and ensure that they are communicating a caring and professional demeanor. Patients may be nervous or anxious about receiving chiropractic treatment, and a reassuring demeanor from the chiropractor can help to put them at ease.

The chiropractic profession has established ethical guidelines to ensure that patients receive safe and effective care. These guidelines include obtaining informed consent, respecting the patient's autonomy, and maintaining patient confidentiality. Chiropractors are also required to maintain accurate and complete patient records and to adhere to all relevant laws and regulations.

In some cases, chiropractic care may not be appropriate for a patient. Chiropractors should be aware of their limitations and refer patients to other health care providers when necessary. This may include referring a patient to a medical doctor for further evaluation or to a physical therapist for additional treatment.

Post-treatment recommendations

Chiropractic care is a non-invasive, holistic approach to healthcare that aims to restore balance to the musculoskeletal and nervous systems. This can be achieved through spinal adjustments, mobilizations, soft tissue techniques, and other therapies. After receiving chiropractic treatment, it is important to follow post-treatment recommendations to maximize the benefits and prevent future problems.

The following are some common post-treatment recommendations that chiropractors may give their patients:

1. Rest and Relaxation: After a chiropractic adjustment, it is important to rest and allow the body to heal. This may mean avoiding strenuous physical activity or exercise for a period of time, as well as getting enough sleep and reducing stress.

2. Ice and Heat Therapy: Depending on the type of treatment received, a chiropractor may recommend the use of ice or heat therapy to reduce pain and inflammation. Ice is typically used for acute injuries or inflammation, while heat is used for chronic pain or stiffness.

3. Stretching and Exercise: Chiropractors may recommend specific stretches or exercises to help maintain the benefits of the treatment and prevent future problems. These exercises may focus on strengthening the core muscles, improving posture, and increasing flexibility.

4. Proper Ergonomics: Chiropractors may also provide recommendations for proper ergonomics to reduce stress on the spine and prevent future in-

juries. This may include adjusting workstation setup, using proper lifting techniques, and maintaining good posture.

5. Hydration and Nutrition: Proper hydration and nutrition are essential for overall health and can also support the body's natural healing process. Chiropractors may recommend drinking plenty of water and eating a balanced diet rich in nutrients and antioxidants.

6. Follow-Up Visits: Depending on the patient's condition and treatment plan, chiropractors may recommend follow-up visits to monitor progress and make adjustments as needed.

It is important for patients to follow these post-treatment recommendations to ensure the best possible outcome from chiropractic care. By taking an active role in their own healthcare, patients can maximize the benefits of chiropractic treatment and improve their overall quality of life.

Chapter Twelve

Chiropractic Myths and Misconceptions

Chiropractic is a form of alternative medicine that is focused on the diagnosis and treatment of neuromuscular disorders, with a particular emphasis on the spine. While chiropractic has been practiced for over a century, there are still many myths and misconceptions surrounding this form of treatment. Below we will explore some of the most common chiropractic myths and misconceptions.

1. Myth #1: Chiropractic is not a real form of medicine

This is one of the most common misconceptions about chiropractic. In fact, chiropractic is a licensed healthcare profession that is recognized in many countries around the world. Chiropractors are trained healthcare professionals who are licensed to diagnose and treat a variety of neuromuscular disorders, with a particular focus on the spine.

2. Myth #2: Chiropractic is only for people with back pain

While chiropractic is often associated with the treatment of back pain, it is actually a very versatile form of treatment that can be used to treat a wide range of conditions. Chiropractors are trained to diagnose and treat a variety of neuromuscular disorders, including neck pain, headaches, and sports injuries.

3. Myth #3: Chiropractic is dangerous

Chiropractic is a safe and effective form of treatment, with a very low risk of complications. In fact, chiropractic is often considered safer than many other forms of medical treatment, including prescription drugs and surgery. However, as with any form of medical treatment, there is always a small risk of complications. Your chiropractor will discuss these risks with you before starting any treatment.

4. Myth #4: Chiropractic is not evidence-based

This is a common misconception that is not supported by the facts. There is a growing body of scientific evidence that supports the use of chiropractic for a variety of neuromuscular disorders. In fact, many medical organizations now recognize chiropractic as a safe and effective form of treatment for conditions such as low back pain and neck pain.

5. Myth #5: Chiropractic is expensive

While it is true that chiropractic treatment can be expensive, it is important to remember that the cost of treatment will vary depending on a number of factors, including the location of the practice and the type of treatment being used. In addition, many health insurance plans now cover chiropractic treatment, which can help to make it more affordable for patients.

6. Myth #6: Chiropractic is not effective

This is another common misconception that is not supported by the facts. There is a growing body of scientific evidence that supports the use of chiropractic for a variety of neuromuscular disorders. In fact, many studies have found that chiropractic is just as effective, if not more effective, than other forms of medical treatment, such as prescription drugs and surgery.

7. Myth #7: Chiropractic treatment is painful

While it is true that some patients may experience mild discomfort or soreness after a chiropractic treatment, this is generally not the case. In fact, most patients find chiropractic treatment to be very comfortable and relaxing. Your chiropractor will work with you to ensure that you are comfortable throughout your treatment.

8. Myth #8: Chiropractors are not real doctors

This is a common misconception that is not supported by the facts. Chiropractors are licensed healthcare professionals who are required to complete a rigorous program of study that is similar in scope to medical school. In addition, chiropractors are required to pass a national board exam in order to become licensed to practice.

Addressing common concerns

Chiropractic care is a complementary healthcare practice that focuses on the diagnosis, treatment, and prevention of musculoskeletal and nervous system disorders. Despite its growing popularity and success in treating various conditions, there are still common concerns and misconceptions surrounding this form of treatment. Below we will address some of the most common concerns and misconceptions about chiropractic care.

One of the most common concerns about chiropractic care is its safety. Some people worry that spinal manipulation, which is a primary treatment technique used by chiropractors, may cause harm or injury. However, studies have shown that chiropractic care is generally safe and effective. In fact, chiropractors undergo extensive training and education to ensure that they can provide safe and effective treatment to their patients. Additionally, chiropractors are trained to recognize any potential risks or contraindications before performing any adjustments or manipulations.

Another concern is that chiropractic care is not supported by scientific evidence. However, numerous studies have demonstrated the effectiveness of chiropractic care in treating a wide range of conditions, including back pain, neck pain, headaches, and musculoskeletal injuries. In fact, the American College of Physicians recommends chiropractic care as a first-line treatment for low back pain.

There is also a misconception that chiropractors only treat back and neck pain. While chiropractors are best known for treating spinal issues, they are trained to address a variety of musculoskeletal and nervous system disorders. Chiropractic care can also help improve posture, alleviate stress and tension, and improve overall health and wellness.

Some people are concerned that chiropractic care is painful or uncomfortable. However, chiropractic adjustments and manipulations are generally painless and often provide immediate relief from pain and discomfort. While some patients may experience mild soreness or discomfort after a treatment, this is usually temporary and dissipates within a few hours to a few days.

Another common misconception is that chiropractic care is not covered by insurance. While insurance coverage for chiropractic care varies depending on the policy and provider, many insurance plans do offer coverage for chiropractic care. Patients are encouraged to check with their insurance provider to determine the extent of their coverage.

Finally, some people believe that chiropractic care is only effective for short-term relief and does not provide long-term benefits. However, numerous studies have demonstrated the long-term effectiveness of chiropractic care for various conditions. Additionally, chiropractors often provide patients with exercises and lifestyle recommendations to help maintain their health and prevent future issues.

Debunking misconceptions

Chiropractic care is a form of alternative medicine that focuses on the relationship between the musculoskeletal system and the nervous system. It involves manual manipulation of the spine and other joints in the body to alleviate pain and improve overall health. Despite its widespread use and proven benefits, chiropractic care is often the subject of misconceptions and myths. Below we will debunk some of the most common misconceptions about chiropractic care.

1. Misconception 1: Chiropractic care is not scientific.

One of the most common misconceptions about chiropractic care is that it is not based on scientific evidence. This is not true. Chiropractic care is a science-based healthcare profession that relies on a deep understanding of the human body, particularly the musculoskeletal and nervous systems. Chiropractors undergo extensive training and education to gain the knowledge and skills required to practice.

Furthermore, there is a growing body of scientific research that supports the effectiveness of chiropractic care for a range of conditions, including back pain, neck pain, headaches, and more. Many studies have shown that chiropractic care can be as effective or even more effective than traditional medical treatments for these conditions.

2. Misconception 2: Chiropractic care is dangerous.

Another common myth about chiropractic care is that it is dangerous and can lead to serious injuries. While it is true that all medical procedures carry some level of risk, chiropractic care is generally considered to be safe when performed by a qualified and experienced practitioner.

The most common side effects of chiropractic care are mild and temporary, such as soreness and stiffness in the treated area. More serious side effects are rare, but they can occur. However, the risk of serious injury from chiropractic care is low, particularly when compared to the risks associated with traditional medical treatments like surgery and medication.

3. Misconception 3: Chiropractic care is not effective.

Another common misconception about chiropractic care is that it is not effective and is only used for back pain. However, this is not true. Chiropractic care has been shown to be effective for a range of conditions, including back pain, neck pain, headaches, sciatica, and more.

In fact, many patients report significant improvement in their symptoms after just a few sessions of chiropractic care. This is because chiropractic care addresses the root cause of many musculoskeletal and nervous system disorders, rather than just treating the symptoms.

4. Misconception 4: Chiropractic care is expensive.

Many people assume that chiropractic care is expensive and not covered by insurance. However, this is not always the case. Many insurance plans, including Medicare and Medicaid, cover chiropractic care. Additionally, many chiropractors offer flexible payment plans and accept various forms of payment, including credit cards and health savings accounts.

Furthermore, chiropractic care can often be more cost-effective than traditional medical treatments, such as surgery and medication, which can be costly and require ongoing treatment. By addressing the root cause of the problem, chiropractic care can often provide long-term relief, saving patients money in the long run.

5. Misconception 5: Chiropractors are not real doctors.

Some people believe that chiropractors are not real doctors and do not have the same level of training and education as medical doctors. However, this is not true. Chiropractors are licensed healthcare professionals who undergo extensive education and training in the diagnosis and treatment of musculoskeletal and nervous system disorders.

Chiropractors must complete a four-year Doctor of Chiropractic program and pass a series of rigorous exams in order to become licensed. They also participate in ongoing education and training to keep their skills and knowledge up-to-date.

Safety and efficacy

Chiropractic is a healthcare profession that emphasizes the diagnosis and treatment of neuromuscular disorders, with a focus on the spine and its relationship to the nervous system. It is a non-invasive and drug-free approach to healthcare that has been gaining in popularity in recent years. Despite its growing popularity, some people still have concerns about the safety and efficacy of chiropractic care. Below we will discuss the safety and efficacy of chiropractic care, debunk some common myths, and provide information to help patients make informed decisions about their healthcare.

Safety

One of the most common concerns people have about chiropractic care is its safety. Some people worry that chiropractic adjustments can cause serious harm or even death. However, research shows that chiropractic care is a safe and effective form of healthcare.

According to a study published in the Journal of Manipulative and Physiological Therapeutics, the risk of serious adverse events following chiropractic care is extremely low. The study found that the incidence of serious adverse events was only one in every five million chiropractic adjustments. To put this in perspective, the risk of serious adverse events following a course of nonsteroidal anti-inflammatory drugs (NSAIDs) is 1 in 1,200.

Chiropractors are highly trained healthcare professionals who undergo rigorous education and training before they are licensed to practice. They must complete a four-year doctoral degree program at an accredited chiropractic college, which includes extensive training in anatomy, physiology, and biomechanics. Chiropractors must also pass a national board exam and obtain a license to practice in their state.

Efficacy

Another concern people have about chiropractic care is its efficacy. Some people believe that chiropractic care is not a valid form of healthcare and that it has no scientific basis. However, research has shown that chiropractic care can be an effective treatment for a variety of musculoskeletal conditions.

For example, a study published in the Annals of Internal Medicine found that chiropractic care was more effective than medication for the treatment of acute low back pain. The study showed that patients who received chiropractic care experienced greater reductions in pain and disability than those who received medication.

Chiropractic care has also been shown to be effective for the treatment of neck pain, headaches, and other musculoskeletal conditions. A study published in the Journal of Manipulative and Physiological Therapeutics found that chiropractic care was effective for the treatment of chronic neck pain. The study showed that patients who received chiropractic care experienced greater reductions in pain and disability than those who received medication.

Debunking Myths

Despite the safety and efficacy of chiropractic care, there are still many myths and misconceptions surrounding this form of healthcare. One common myth is that chiropractic care is only effective for the treatment of back pain. However, chiropractic care has been shown to be effective for a variety of musculoskeletal conditions, including neck pain, headaches, and joint pain.

Another myth is that chiropractic care is not based on scientific evidence. However, chiropractic care is based on the scientific principles of anatomy, physiology, and biomechanics. Chiropractors use evidence-based treatments that have been shown to be effective for the treatment of musculoskeletal conditions.

Addressing Concerns

If you have concerns about chiropractic care, it is important to talk to your chiropractor. Your chiropractor can provide you with information about the safety and efficacy of chiropractic care and address any concerns you may have. They can also provide you with information about the risks and benefits of chiropractic care and help you make an informed decision about your healthcare.

It is also important to choose a licensed and qualified chiropractor. Look for a chiropractor who has completed a four-year doctoral degree program at an accredited chiropractic college and who has passed a national board

Chapter Thirteen

Chiropractic Research and Evidence

Chiropractic is a complementary and alternative medicine (CAM) therapy that focuses on diagnosing and treating disorders of the musculoskeletal system, particularly the spine. It has been gaining popularity over the past few decades, with millions of people seeking chiropractic care each year. However, like any form of medical treatment, the safety and efficacy of chiropractic care are often called into question, and it is important to explore the research and evidence behind it.

One of the main criticisms of chiropractic care is the lack of scientific evidence supporting its effectiveness. While some studies have suggested that chiropractic can be effective in treating certain musculoskeletal conditions such as lower back pain, neck pain, and headaches, the quality of the research is often criticized. Many studies suffer from small sample sizes, lack of control groups, and other methodological issues that make it difficult to draw strong conclusions.

Despite these challenges, there is a growing body of evidence that suggests that chiropractic can be an effective treatment for certain conditions. For example, a 2017 study published in the Journal of the American Medical Association found that chiropractic care, in combination with usual medical care, can help reduce lower back pain more effectively than usual medical care alone. Another study published in the Journal of Manipulative and Physiological Therapeutics found that chiropractic care can be an effective treatment for chronic neck pain.

In addition to these studies, there are also many anecdotal reports from patients who have experienced significant relief from their symptoms after receiving chiropractic care. While anecdotal evidence is not the same as scientific evidence, it can still provide valuable insights into the potential benefits of chiropractic care.

One of the reasons why chiropractic care is often criticized is that it is based on a theory of subluxations, which are said to be misalignments of the vertebrae that interfere with nerve function and cause a variety of health problems. While the existence of subluxations has been questioned by many medical professionals, there is evidence to suggest that chiropractic adjustments can have a positive impact on the nervous system.

For example, a study published in the Journal of Manipulative and Physiological Therapeutics found that chiropractic adjustments can help improve the function of the autonomic nervous system, which is responsible for regulating many of the body's automatic functions such as heart rate, digestion, and breathing. Another study published in the Journal of Alternative and Complementary Medicine found that chiropractic adjustments can help increase the production of antibodies in the body, which can help boost the immune system.

It is also important to note that chiropractic care is generally considered to be safe, with few serious side effects reported. However, like any medical treatment, there are some risks associated with chiropractic care, particularly if the treatment is not performed correctly or by a qualified practitioner. These risks can include nerve damage, stroke, and other serious complications.

Current studies and findings

Chiropractic is a healthcare profession that focuses on the diagnosis, treatment, and prevention of disorders of the musculoskeletal system, particularly the spine. It is a non-invasive, drug-free approach to health care that utilizes a variety of techniques, including spinal adjustments, to improve the function of the nervous system and the body as a whole. The effectiveness of chiropractic care has been a topic of debate in the medical community, and many studies have been conducted to determine its safety and efficacy.

Current studies have shown that chiropractic care can be effective in treating a wide range of musculoskeletal conditions, including neck pain, back pain, and headaches. One study published in the Annals of Internal Medicine found that spinal manipulation was effective in relieving acute low back pain, with improvements in pain and function lasting up to six weeks. Another study published in the Journal of Manipulative and Physiological Therapeutics found that chiropractic care was effective in reducing neck pain, with patients reporting a significant decrease in pain and improvement in function.

Research has also shown that chiropractic care can be effective in treating other conditions, such as carpal tunnel syndrome, fibromyalgia, and sciatica. One study published in the Journal of Chiropractic Medicine found that chiropractic care was effective in reducing pain and improving grip strength in patients with carpal tunnel syndrome. Another study published in the Journal of Alternative and Complementary Medicine found that chiropractic care was effective in reducing pain and improving quality of life in patients with fibromyalgia.

In addition to musculoskeletal conditions, chiropractic care may also be beneficial for other health conditions. One study published in the Journal of Manipulative and Physiological Therapeutics found that chiropractic care was effective in reducing the frequency and intensity of migraines in patients who received regular chiropractic adjustments. Another study published in the Journal of Chiropractic Medicine found that chiropractic care was effective in reducing blood pressure in patients with hypertension.

While many studies have shown the effectiveness of chiropractic care, it is important to note that not all studies have produced positive results. One study published in the Journal of the American Medical Association found that chiropractic care was no more effective than traditional medical care in treating acute low back pain. However, it is important to note that this study only looked at a specific type of chiropractic manipulation, and other techniques may be more effective.

Despite the mixed results of some studies, the overall evidence suggests that chiropractic care is a safe and effective treatment option for a variety of musculoskeletal conditions. Chiropractors undergo extensive training and are licensed healthcare professionals who are trained to diagnose and treat musculoskeletal conditions. They use a variety of techniques, including spinal adjustments, to help patients achieve optimal health and wellness.

Efficacy for various conditions

Chiropractic is a healthcare profession that focuses on the diagnosis, treatment, and prevention of musculoskeletal disorders, particularly those related to the spine. Chiropractors use a range of techniques, including spinal manipulation, to help alleviate pain, improve mobility, and promote overall health and wellbeing. Over the years, chiropractic care has gained popularity as an alternative or complementary treatment to traditional medical approaches. Research has been conducted to evaluate the efficacy of chiropractic care for various conditions, and the results have been promising.

Low Back Pain

Low back pain is one of the most common reasons people seek chiropractic care. A systematic review of randomized controlled trials (RCTs) found that spinal manipulation was associated with statistically significant improvements in pain and function for patients with acute low back pain compared to sham manipulation or other interventions. Similarly, a meta-analysis of RCTs found that spinal manipulation was effective in reducing pain and improving function for patients with chronic low back pain, with effects comparable to other commonly used treatments like exercise and nonsteroidal anti-inflammatory drugs (NSAIDs).

Neck Pain

Neck pain is another common complaint for which patients seek chiropractic care. A 2017 study published in the Annals of Internal Medicine found that chiropractic care, specifically spinal manipulation and mobilization, was more effective than medication in reducing pain for patients with acute neck pain. Additionally, a systematic review of RCTs found that spinal manipulation was associated with moderate to large short-term improvements in pain and function for patients with chronic neck pain.

Headaches

Headaches are a frequent complaint for which patients seek chiropractic care. A 2011 systematic review of RCTs found that spinal manipulation was effective in reducing the frequency and intensity of migraines and tension-type headaches. Another review of the literature found that chiropractic care was more effective than placebo or other interventions in reducing headache pain, with effects lasting up to six months.

Sports Injuries

Chiropractic care has been shown to be effective in the treatment of sports injuries. A review of the literature found that chiropractic care was effective in treating common musculoskeletal injuries like ankle sprains, plantar fasciitis, and patellofemoral pain syndrome. Additionally, a case series found that chiropractic care was effective in improving ankle range of motion and reducing pain for professional football players.

Pediatrics

Chiropractic care is often sought for pediatric patients as well. A systematic review of the literature found that chiropractic care was safe and effective in the treatment of various pediatric conditions, including musculoskeletal pain, asthma, otitis media, and colic. Additionally, a case series found that chiropractic care was effective in reducing the frequency and severity of ear infections in pediatric patients.

Future research directions

Chiropractic care has been around for over a century, and it continues to evolve as research advances. Over the years, numerous studies have been conducted to assess the effectiveness of chiropractic care in treating various conditions. While chiropractic care is most commonly associated with treating back and neck pain, studies have explored its efficacy for other conditions such as headaches, migraines, sports injuries, and even prenatal care.

Despite the significant progress in the field of chiropractic research, there is still much to be learned about the practice. Future research directions aim to address the gaps in our current understanding of chiropractic care and explore how it can be incorporated into mainstream healthcare.

One area of future research is the exploration of the mechanisms of action underlying chiropractic care. Despite the widespread use of chiropractic care, the precise mechanisms of action that underlie the benefits of spinal manipulation remain unclear. Some theories suggest that spinal manipulation may affect the nervous system, while others suggest that it may alter blood flow and circulation. Further research is needed to clarify the underlying mechanisms of action and how they contribute to the therapeutic benefits of chiropractic care.

Another area of future research is the exploration of the effectiveness of chiropractic care for various populations. While chiropractic care is commonly used among adults, there is limited research on its effectiveness for children, seniors, and pregnant women. Future research in this area could help identify the potential benefits and risks of chiropractic care for different populations, as well as develop specialized techniques and approaches to meet their unique needs.

Furthermore, future research can also focus on identifying and measuring the long-term effects of chiropractic care. While many studies have evaluated the short-term effects of chiropractic care, few have examined the long-term effects. Understanding the long-term effects of chiropractic care can help us determine the most effective treatment strategies and develop preventive measures to reduce the risk of future injuries.

Additionally, future research can explore how chiropractic care can be integrated into mainstream healthcare. Chiropractic care has traditionally been viewed as an alternative form of healthcare. However, as more research highlights the potential benefits of chiropractic care, there is increasing interest in incorporating it into mainstream healthcare. Future research can explore how chiropractic care can be integrated into conventional healthcare models to provide patients with a comprehensive and holistic approach to healthcare.

Lastly, future research can explore the effectiveness of various chiropractic techniques and approaches. While spinal manipulation is the most commonly used chiropractic technique, there are other techniques such as mobilization, soft tissue techniques, and instrument-assisted techniques. Furthermore, chiropractors may also use different approaches such as the Gonstead technique or the Activator method. Further research is needed to determine the effectiveness of these techniques and approaches for different conditions and patient populations.

Chapter Fourteen

Chiropractic Ethics and Professionalism

Chiropractic care is a profession that requires high levels of professionalism and ethics to ensure the safety and well-being of patients. Professionalism and ethics in chiropractic practice are crucial because chiropractors often work closely with vulnerable individuals, including those with musculoskeletal disorders, back pain, and other conditions. As such, chiropractors are responsible for providing quality and ethical care to all their patients. Below we will explore the importance of ethics and professionalism in chiropractic practice, as well as the guidelines and standards that chiropractors must follow to ensure safe and effective patient care.

Ethics in chiropractic care refers to the moral principles and values that govern the behavior of chiropractors. Ethics are important in chiropractic practice because they help to establish trust between the patient and the chiropractor, ensuring that the patient receives the best possible care. One of the primary ethical responsibilities of chiropractors is to obtain informed consent from their patients before providing any treatment. Informed consent means that the patient understands the nature of the treatment, its potential benefits and risks, and any alternatives that may be available. Chiropractors must also respect the confidentiality and privacy of their patients and maintain accurate records of all treatments provided.

Another essential aspect of chiropractic ethics is the duty to provide competent and safe care to patients. Chiropractors must maintain high levels of knowledge and skill through ongoing education and training to ensure that they provide the most effective and safe care possible. They must also practice within their scope of competence and refer patients to other healthcare professionals when necessary.

Professionalism in chiropractic care refers to the behaviors and attitudes that chiropractors exhibit in their interactions with patients, other healthcare professionals, and the public. Professionalism is essential because it helps to build trust, respect, and credibility between the chiropractor and their patients, and it enhances the reputation of the chiropractic profession as a whole. Chiropractors must display a high level of professionalism by being honest, transparent, and respectful in all their interactions with patients.

Chiropractors must also adhere to a strict code of ethics and professional conduct established by the chiropractic profession's governing bodies. For example, the International Chiropractors Association (ICA) has established a Code of Ethics that outlines the ethical responsibilities of chiropractors. The code includes guidelines for informed consent, confidentiality, competence, advertising, and research. Chiropractors who violate the code of ethics may face disciplinary action, including the loss of their license to practice.

Chiropractors must also follow the standards and guidelines set by the regulatory bodies that govern the chiropractic profession. For example, in the United States, chiropractors must be licensed by the state in which they practice, and they must meet the education and training requirements established by the National Board of Chiropractic Examiners (NBCE). The NBCE sets the standards for chiropractic education, including the minimum number of hours of classroom instruction and clinical experience required.

In addition to the ethical and professional standards outlined above, chiropractors must also be aware of the legal and regulatory requirements that govern their practice. For example, they must comply with federal and state laws related to patient privacy and data security, as well as regulations related to billing and insurance. Chiropractors must also obtain malpractice insurance to protect themselves and their patients in case of a lawsuit.

Code of ethics

Chiropractic is a profession that focuses on the diagnosis, treatment, and prevention of musculoskeletal disorders, particularly those involving the spine. As with any healthcare profession, chiropractors must adhere to a code of ethics to ensure that they provide safe and effective care to their patients. Below we will explore the code of ethics that chiropractors must follow and why it is important.

The code of ethics for chiropractors is designed to promote the highest standards of professional conduct, protect patients' rights and interests, and maintain the integrity and reputation of the profession. The code outlines the ethical principles that chiropractors should follow in their interactions with patients, colleagues, and the public.

One of the most important principles outlined in the code of ethics is the duty of care. Chiropractors have a duty to act in the best interests of their patients and provide care that is safe, effective, and appropriate for their condition. This duty includes a responsibility to obtain informed consent from patients before providing any treatment and to ensure that patients are fully aware of the risks and benefits of the treatment.

Another important principle in the code of ethics is professionalism. Chiropractors are expected to maintain high standards of professionalism in their interactions with patients, colleagues, and the public. This includes demonstrating integrity, honesty, and respect for others at all times, and avoiding any conduct that could harm the reputation of the profession.

The code of ethics also emphasizes the importance of ongoing professional development. Chiropractors are encouraged to engage in continuing education and to stay up-to-date with the latest research and developments in the field. This helps to ensure that they are providing the best possible care to their patients and maintaining the highest standards of professional conduct.

In addition to the code of ethics, chiropractors are also subject to a range of laws and regulations that govern their practice. These include regulations around the use of diagnostic imaging, the prescribing of medication, and the provision of care to minors and vulnerable adults. Chiropractors must also adhere to laws around advertising and marketing, and must ensure that they are providing accurate and truthful information to their patients and the public.

The code of ethics for chiropractors is an important tool for ensuring that patients receive safe, effective, and ethical care. By adhering to these principles, chiropractors can build trust with their patients and the wider community, and maintain the integrity and reputation of the profession. Patients can feel confident that they are receiving care from a qualified and ethical practitioner, and can be assured that their interests and rights are being protected.

Patient rights and responsibilities

Chiropractic care has become a popular alternative healthcare option for many people who want to improve their musculoskeletal health and overall well-being. Chiropractors are trained to diagnose and treat conditions that affect the body's musculoskeletal system, primarily the spine. While chiropractic care is generally safe and effective, patients also have rights and responsibilities that must be respected and followed for a successful outcome.

One of the most important patient rights is the right to informed consent. Informed consent is the process of providing patients with information about the proposed treatment, including the risks, benefits, and alternatives, so they can make an informed decision about their care. It is the chiropractor's responsibility to explain the diagnosis, treatment plan, and any potential side effects to the patient before beginning treatment.

Patients also have the right to refuse treatment or ask for a second opinion. Chiropractors should respect their patients' decisions and provide them with alternative treatment options if available. If a patient does not understand something, they should ask for clarification until they are comfortable with the proposed treatment.

In addition to informed consent, patients also have responsibilities in chiropractic care. Patients must provide complete and accurate medical histories, including any medications they are taking, past surgeries, or any other relevant health information. This information can help chiropractors make informed decisions about the appropriate treatment plan.

Patients should also follow the treatment plan as prescribed by the chiropractor, attend all scheduled appointments, and provide feedback on how the treatment is affecting their condition. If a patient experiences any adverse effects or discomfort during treatment, they should inform the chiropractor immediately.

Another important aspect of patient rights in chiropractic care is confidentiality. Chiropractors must maintain strict confidentiality of patient information, including medical records, diagnosis, and treatment plans.

Patients can trust that their personal and health information will not be disclosed without their written consent.

Along with patient rights and responsibilities, it is also important to understand the ethical principles and standards of professional conduct that guide chiropractors. The American Chiropractic Association has established a code of ethics that all chiropractors must follow.

The code of ethics covers several areas, including the chiropractor's responsibility to provide competent care, maintain professional boundaries, and respect the patient's dignity and rights. It also outlines the chiropractor's obligation to maintain confidentiality, obtain informed consent, and refer patients to other healthcare professionals when appropriate.

Chiropractors are also held to high standards of professionalism, including honesty, integrity, and accountability. They must maintain accurate and complete patient records, provide appropriate referrals when necessary, and continually update their knowledge and skills through continuing education.

Continuing education and professional development

Chiropractic is a profession that requires continuous education and professional development to ensure that chiropractors are up-to-date with the latest research and techniques in the field. Below we will explore the importance of continuing education and professional development for chiropractors.

Continuing education is the process of acquiring new knowledge, skills, and competencies beyond the basic education required for licensure. In the United States, chiropractors are required to complete continuing education credits to maintain their licensure. These credits may be obtained through attending seminars, workshops, online courses, and other educational activities.

One of the main reasons for continuing education is to ensure that chiropractors are providing the highest quality of care to their patients. By staying up-to-date with the latest research and techniques in the field, chiropractors can provide better treatment options and outcomes for their patients. For example, if a new technique or technology is developed that has been proven to be effective in treating a certain condition, a chiropractor who has completed continuing education on this topic will be able to offer this treatment option to their patients.

Another benefit of continuing education is that it helps chiropractors to stay current with changes in the healthcare industry. The healthcare industry is constantly evolving, with new regulations, laws, and guidelines being introduced on a regular basis. By staying informed of these changes, chiropractors can ensure that they are providing care that is compliant with current standards and regulations.

Continuing education also provides an opportunity for chiropractors to network with their peers and colleagues in the field. By attending seminars and workshops, chiropractors can connect with others who share their interests and passion for the field. This can lead to collaborations and partnerships that can benefit both the chiropractors and their patients.

Professional development is another important aspect of chiropractic practice. This involves developing skills and competencies that are relevant to the profession, such as communication skills, business management, and leadership skills. Professional development can be achieved through attending workshops and seminars, working with a mentor, or pursuing additional education.

One of the benefits of professional development is that it can enhance the chiropractor's career opportunities. By developing a wide range of skills and competencies, chiropractors can expand their practice and take on new roles within the healthcare industry. For example, a chiropractor who has developed strong leadership and management skills may be able to take on a role as a clinic director or practice owner.

Another benefit of professional development is that it can improve patient care. By developing strong communication skills, chiropractors can better understand their patients' needs and concerns, and provide more effective treatment options. Similarly, by developing business management skills, chiropractors can ensure that their practice is efficient and effective, which can lead to better patient outcomes.

Chapter Fifteen

The Future of Chiropractic

The practice of chiropractic has been around for over a century, and in that time, it has evolved and changed significantly. Today, chiropractic care is a widely recognized and respected form of healthcare, with millions of people around the world seeking treatment from chiropractors for a variety of conditions. As we look to the future of chiropractic, it is clear that this field will continue to grow and evolve in exciting new ways.

One of the most significant trends in the chiropractic field today is the emphasis on evidence-based care. As the scientific community continues to conduct research into the effectiveness of chiropractic treatments, we are seeing more and more evidence that chiropractic care can be an effective treatment for a wide range of conditions. This evidence-based approach to care is helping to legitimize the field of chiropractic and is making it easier for patients to receive the care they need.

Another trend that is shaping the future of chiropractic is the integration of technology into chiropractic practice. Today, there are many advanced diagnostic tools and treatment modalities that chiropractors can use to help their patients. For example, chiropractors can use digital X-rays to diagnose conditions, and they can use laser therapy to help speed up the healing process. As technology continues to advance, we can expect to see even more innovative treatments and diagnostic tools being developed for use in chiropractic care.

One area where we are already seeing significant growth in the chiropractic field is in the use of telehealth. With the rise of telemedicine, it is now possible for patients to receive chiropractic care from the comfort of their own homes. This is especially important for patients who live in remote areas or who have mobility issues that make it difficult for them to travel to a chiropractor's office. As telehealth technology continues to improve, we can expect to see more and more patients seeking chiropractic care online.

Another trend that is shaping the future of chiropractic is the increasing emphasis on wellness and prevention. Chiropractors have long recognized the importance of preventative care in maintaining overall health and wellness, and today, there is a growing focus on educating patients about the importance of lifestyle factors like diet and exercise. By taking a proactive approach to healthcare, chiropractors can help their patients avoid many common health problems and maintain optimal health and wellness throughout their lives.

Of course, with any evolving field, there are also challenges that must be addressed. One of the biggest challenges facing the chiropractic field today is the issue of scope of practice. In some states and countries, chiropractors are not allowed to perform certain procedures or provide certain types of care, which can limit their ability to provide the best possible care to their patients. As the field of chiropractic continues to evolve, it will be important to address these issues and work to ensure that chiropractors are able to provide the highest quality care to their patients.

Innovations and advancements

Chiropractic is a field of healthcare that focuses on the diagnosis and treatment of neuromuscular disorders, with a primary emphasis on manual adjustment and manipulation of the spine. It is a non-invasive, drug-free approach that has gained popularity in recent years as an alternative or complementary treatment option to traditional medical care.

As with many healthcare fields, chiropractic is constantly evolving and adapting to new advancements and innovations in technology and research. Below we will explore some of the most exciting and promising innovations and advancements in chiropractic care.

One of the most significant advancements in chiropractic care in recent years is the increasing use of technology to improve diagnosis and treatment outcomes. One such innovation is the use of digital radiography, which allows chiropractors to obtain more precise and detailed images of the spine and other areas of the body, leading to more accurate diagnosis and treatment plans. Another emerging technology is the use of telehealth, which allows patients to receive virtual consultations and treatment from the comfort of their own homes.

Another promising advancement in chiropractic care is the increasing recognition of the importance of a holistic approach to healthcare. This approach takes into account not just the physical symptoms of a patient, but also their emotional, mental, and social well-being. Many chiropractors are now incorporating mindfulness practices, nutrition counseling, and other lifestyle interventions into their treatment plans to provide a more comprehensive and individualized approach to care.

In addition to technological advancements and a more holistic approach, there are also exciting developments in the research surrounding chiropractic care. One recent study published in the Journal of Manipulative and Physiological Therapeutics found that chiropractic care was effective in reducing pain and disability in patients with chronic low back pain. Another study published in the Journal of Alternative and Complementary

Medicine found that chiropractic care was effective in reducing symptoms of tension headaches.

There are also several ongoing research projects exploring the potential benefits of chiropractic care for a range of other conditions, including asthma, carpal tunnel syndrome, and even some neurological disorders. As the research continues to evolve and expand, it is likely that chiropractic care will become an increasingly recognized and accepted form of healthcare.

Finally, the future of chiropractic care also lies in the hands of the next generation of chiropractors. As more and more students enter chiropractic schools, there is a growing emphasis on interprofessional education and collaboration with other healthcare providers. This collaboration not only helps to ensure that patients receive the most comprehensive and effective care possible, but also helps to break down traditional barriers and misconceptions between different healthcare fields.

Integrating technology

Chiropractic care is a form of healthcare that focuses on the diagnosis and treatment of musculoskeletal disorders, especially those related to the spine. Over the years, chiropractors have been at the forefront of using innovative and advanced technologies to improve patient outcomes. Technology has enabled chiropractors to provide more accurate diagnoses, target treatment to specific areas, and improve patient communication and engagement. Below we will discuss some of the latest technological advancements that are being used in chiropractic care.

Digital Imaging:

Digital imaging is a non-invasive diagnostic tool that uses digital technology to produce high-quality images of the spine and surrounding areas. Digital X-rays, CT scans, and MRI scans are all examples of digital imaging techniques that are commonly used in chiropractic care. Digital imaging has several advantages over traditional imaging techniques. For example, digital X-rays use less radiation than traditional X-rays and produce images that can be viewed immediately, reducing the need for repeat X-rays. Additionally, digital imaging allows chiropractors to share images with other healthcare providers, which can be especially helpful in complex cases.

Electrodiagnostic Testing:

Electrodiagnostic testing is a type of diagnostic tool that measures the electrical activity of muscles and nerves. This test can help chiropractors identify nerve damage or other underlying conditions that may be contributing to a patient's symptoms. Electromyography (EMG) and nerve conduction velocity (NCV) tests are examples of electrodiagnostic tests that are commonly used in chiropractic care.

Infrared Thermography:

Infrared thermography is a non-invasive diagnostic tool that uses infrared technology to detect temperature changes in the body. This technique can be used to identify areas of inflammation or nerve dysfunction, which can help chiropractors target treatment more effectively. Infrared thermography is particularly useful in treating conditions such as whiplash, where underlying soft tissue damage can be difficult to diagnose.

Pulsed Electromagnetic Field Therapy:

Pulsed electromagnetic field therapy (PEMF) is a type of therapy that uses electromagnetic fields to stimulate healing in damaged tissues. PEMF therapy has been shown to be effective in reducing inflammation, increasing blood flow, and promoting tissue repair. It is often used in conjunction with chiropractic adjustments to enhance the effects of the adjustment and promote healing.

Computerized Adjustment Instruments:

Computerized adjustment instruments are advanced tools that use technology to deliver precise, targeted adjustments to the spine. These instruments are particularly useful in treating patients with complex conditions or injuries. For example, a computerized instrument can be used to adjust specific vertebrae in the spine without putting pressure on surrounding areas. This can be especially helpful in treating conditions such as herniated discs, where precision is critical.

Telehealth:

Telehealth is a technology-based service that allows patients to receive care from their chiropractor remotely. This service is particularly useful for patients who are unable to visit their chiropractor in person due to distance, mobility issues, or other health concerns. Telehealth services can include video consultations, virtual check-ins, and remote monitoring of patient progress. Telehealth has become increasingly important during the COVID-19 pandemic, as it allows chiropractors to continue providing care to patients while minimizing the risk of exposure.

Expanding the scope of practice

Chiropractic care has been growing in popularity and recognition over the years due to its effectiveness in treating various musculoskeletal conditions. In recent times, there has been a growing movement to expand the scope of practice of chiropractors, allowing them to treat a wider range of health conditions. This has led to debates and discussions about the safety and efficacy of these expanded services.

Traditionally, chiropractic care has been focused on the diagnosis, treatment, and prevention of conditions related to the musculoskeletal system, particularly the spine. This includes conditions such as back pain, neck pain, headaches, and other related issues. Chiropractors use a variety of techniques, such as spinal adjustments, mobilization, and soft tissue therapy, to help alleviate pain and improve the function of the affected area.

However, there is growing interest in expanding the scope of chiropractic practice to include other areas of healthcare, such as primary care, sports medicine, and nutrition. Many chiropractors believe that they are well-equipped to provide these services, as they have a holistic approach to healthcare and are trained to consider the whole body rather than just individual symptoms.

One area where chiropractors are increasingly involved is in the management of chronic pain. Chronic pain is a complex and multifaceted condition that can be challenging to treat. Chiropractors have expertise in managing musculoskeletal pain, and there is growing evidence to support the use of chiropractic care as part of a multidisciplinary approach to managing chronic pain.

Chiropractors are also becoming more involved in sports medicine. They are well-equipped to provide pre- and post-game treatments, as well as rehabilitation for sports injuries. Chiropractic care can help athletes recover from injuries faster and improve their overall performance.

Another area where chiropractors are expanding their scope of practice is in nutrition. Many chiropractors recognize the importance of proper nutrition in maintaining good health and preventing chronic disease. They can provide patients with advice and guidance on healthy eating habits, supplementation, and other related topics.

However, the expansion of chiropractic care into these areas has led to some controversy. Some critics argue that chiropractors do not have the necessary training or qualifications to provide these services safely and effectively. There are also concerns that chiropractors may be overstepping their scope of practice and potentially putting patients at risk.

To address these concerns, chiropractors must ensure that they have the necessary qualifications and training to provide expanded services safely and effectively. This may involve obtaining additional certifications, completing additional training programs, or collaborating with other healthcare professionals to provide a multidisciplinary approach to patient care.

Chapter Sixteen

Chiropractic for Athletes

Chiropractic is a healthcare profession that focuses on the diagnosis and treatment of musculoskeletal and nervous system disorders, especially those related to the spine. Chiropractic has been gaining popularity among athletes because of its non-invasive and drug-free approach to treating sports injuries and improving athletic performance.

Athletes, both professional and amateur, are prone to injuries due to the physical demands of their sport. These injuries can cause pain, inflammation, restricted movement, and decreased performance. Chiropractic care can help athletes recover from injuries, prevent future injuries, and enhance their overall performance.

One of the primary benefits of chiropractic care for athletes is pain relief. Chiropractors use various techniques, such as spinal adjustments, soft tissue mobilization, and stretching, to alleviate pain and inflammation caused by injuries. By reducing pain and inflammation, chiropractic care can help athletes return to their sport sooner and perform at a higher level.

Chiropractic care can also help athletes prevent injuries by improving their biomechanics and posture. Chiropractors can identify and correct imbalances in the spine and joints that can lead to overuse injuries. By improving joint mobility and range of motion, chiropractic care can also help athletes move more efficiently and reduce the risk of injury.

In addition to treating injuries and preventing future ones, chiropractic care can also enhance athletic performance. Chiropractors can improve an athlete's overall flexibility, balance, and coordination, which are essential for many sports. By improving an athlete's body mechanics, chiropractic care can also help them generate more power and speed, leading to better performance.

Chiropractors also work closely with other healthcare professionals, such as sports medicine physicians and physical therapists, to provide comprehensive care to athletes. By collaborating with other healthcare providers, chiropractors can ensure that athletes receive the most appropriate and effective care for their injuries.

Another benefit of chiropractic care for athletes is that it is non-invasive and drug-free. Unlike many traditional medical treatments for sports injuries, chiropractic care does not involve surgery or prescription medication. Chiropractors use natural, non-invasive techniques to treat injuries and enhance athletic performance, making it a safer and healthier option for athletes.

When seeking chiropractic care for sports injuries, it is essential to find a chiropractor who specializes in working with athletes. These chiropractors have advanced training and experience in treating sports injuries and working with athletes of all levels. They can also provide customized treatment plans that address the unique needs and goals of each athlete.

Performance enhancement

Chiropractic care has become increasingly popular among athletes who seek to enhance their performance and prevent injuries. Chiropractors use non-invasive techniques to restore and maintain the musculoskeletal system's function and balance, helping athletes improve their overall physical abilities.

Chiropractic care can benefit athletes in several ways, including:

1. Pain Relief: Chiropractors use spinal adjustments and other techniques to alleviate pain caused by injuries, muscle strains, and other conditions. This allows athletes to recover faster and get back to training and competition sooner.

2. Improved Flexibility: Chiropractors can help athletes improve their range of motion, which can help them perform better and reduce the risk of injuries.

3. Enhanced Strength: Chiropractors can help athletes build strength by using techniques like spinal manipulation, massage therapy, and exercise therapy.

4. Improved Balance: Chiropractors can help athletes improve their balance and coordination, which can help prevent injuries.

5. Faster Recovery: Chiropractic care can help athletes recover faster from injuries and reduce the risk of future injuries.

6. Increased Endurance: Chiropractic care can help athletes increase their endurance by reducing pain, improving flexibility, and enhancing overall physical performance.

Chiropractors also work with athletes to develop personalized treatment plans that take into account their specific needs and goals. This can include recommendations for nutrition, exercise, and other lifestyle changes that can help athletes achieve their performance goals.

In addition to providing care for individual athletes, chiropractors can also work with sports teams and organizations to promote overall health and wellness. This can include providing education and training on injury prevention, nutrition, and other topics related to sports performance.

Chiropractors can also work in conjunction with other healthcare providers, such as physical therapists, athletic trainers, and sports medicine doctors, to provide comprehensive care for athletes.

Chiropractic care has been shown to be safe and effective for athletes of all levels, from amateurs to professionals. Studies have found that chiropractic care can improve athletic performance, reduce the risk of injuries, and improve overall health and wellness.

In one study, college football players who received chiropractic care for their injuries were found to have a faster recovery time and a lower risk of reinjury compared to those who did not receive chiropractic care.

In another study, professional basketball players who received chiropractic care reported improved range of motion, flexibility, and overall physical performance.

Injury prevention

Injury prevention is a vital aspect of sports and athletics, as injuries can significantly impact an athlete's performance, leading to reduced training time and potential long-term damage. Chiropractic care can play a crucial role in injury prevention by helping athletes maintain proper alignment, range of motion, and overall body mechanics. Below we will discuss how chiropractic care can help prevent injuries in athletes.

Chiropractors use various techniques to assess an athlete's musculoskeletal system, identifying any imbalances or restrictions that may affect their performance or lead to injuries. For example, they may use motion analysis software to identify movement patterns that may lead to injuries or evaluate joint mobility to identify any restrictions that may lead to compensations in other areas of the body.

One technique commonly used by chiropractors to prevent injuries is spinal manipulation, also known as an adjustment. Spinal manipulation involves applying controlled force to a joint to improve its range of motion and restore proper alignment. By improving spinal mobility, athletes can better absorb shock and stress during athletic activities, reducing the risk of injury.

Chiropractors may also use soft tissue techniques, such as massage or stretching, to improve muscle function and flexibility. These techniques can help athletes avoid overuse injuries by reducing tension in muscles and promoting healthy blood flow.

In addition to physical techniques, chiropractors may also provide advice on nutrition and supplementation to support optimal athletic performance and prevent injuries. For example, they may recommend specific nutrients or supplements to support bone health, reduce inflammation, and improve recovery time.

Chiropractors also work with athletes to improve their overall body mechanics and movement patterns. By assessing an athlete's gait, posture, and other movements, chiropractors can identify areas of weakness or imbalance that may increase the risk of injury. They may then provide corrective exercises or recommend changes to an athlete's training regimen to address these issues and prevent injuries.

Athletes who receive chiropractic care regularly can benefit from improved joint mobility, increased flexibility, reduced tension and inflammation, and improved overall body mechanics. These benefits can help athletes prevent injuries and perform at their best.

It is important to note that chiropractic care should be integrated into a comprehensive sports injury prevention program, including appropriate training, nutrition, and rest. Chiropractic care should not be used as a replacement for other medical treatments, such as physical therapy or surgery, when necessary.

Recovery and rehabilitation

Chiropractic care has become increasingly popular among athletes as a safe and effective way to treat and prevent injuries, as well as aid in recovery and rehabilitation. Chiropractors work with athletes of all levels, from amateur to professional, in a variety of sports, including football, basketball, soccer, hockey, and many others. Below we will explore the benefits of chiropractic care for athletes, with a focus on recovery and rehabilitation.

Chiropractic care is a form of healthcare that focuses on the diagnosis, treatment, and prevention of musculoskeletal disorders, particularly those related to the spine. Chiropractors use hands-on techniques, such as spinal manipulation and mobilization, to relieve pain, reduce inflammation, and restore function. These techniques can also help to improve joint mobility, muscle strength, and overall physical performance.

For athletes, chiropractic care can be particularly beneficial in the recovery and rehabilitation process following an injury. Injuries are a common occurrence in sports, and they can range from minor sprains and strains to more serious conditions such as torn ligaments or fractured bones. Chiropractic care can help to speed up the healing process and reduce the risk of further injury.

One of the primary benefits of chiropractic care for athletes is its ability to reduce pain and inflammation. Pain is a common symptom of many sports injuries, and it can be debilitating, affecting an athlete's ability to perform at their best. Chiropractic care can help to reduce pain and inflammation through spinal manipulation and other manual therapies, such as massage and stretching.

Chiropractic care can also help to improve joint mobility, which is essential for athletes in order to perform at their best. Joint mobility is the ability of a joint to move through its full range of motion, and it is essential for proper movement and athletic performance. Chiropractors can use manual therapies to improve joint mobility and reduce stiffness, allowing athletes to move more freely and with greater ease.

In addition to reducing pain and improving joint mobility, chiropractic care can also help to prevent future injuries. Chiropractors can work with athletes to identify areas of weakness or imbalance in the body and develop a treatment plan to address these issues. This may include exercises to strengthen weak muscles or stretches to improve flexibility and range of motion. By addressing these issues, chiropractors can help to reduce the risk of future injuries and improve overall physical performance.

Chiropractic care can also be a valuable tool in the rehabilitation process following an injury. Rehabilitation is a critical component of the recovery process, as it involves restoring function and range of motion to the injured area. Chiropractors can work with athletes to develop a rehabilitation plan that includes manual therapies, exercises, and other techniques to help speed up the healing process and improve overall function.

Chapter Seventeen

The Role of Chiropractic in Pain Management

The role of chiropractic in pain management has been the subject of much discussion and research in recent years. Chiropractic care is an alternative to traditional medical treatments for pain, offering patients a non-invasive, drug-free approach to managing and relieving pain. Below we will explore the benefits of chiropractic care for pain management and its effectiveness as a treatment option.

Chiropractic care is based on the idea that the body has an innate ability to heal itself. Chiropractors work to facilitate this healing process by adjusting the spine and other joints to relieve pain and improve function. The primary goal of chiropractic care is to alleviate pain and improve the overall health of patients.

One of the primary benefits of chiropractic care is its non-invasive nature. Unlike surgery or other invasive medical procedures, chiropractic care is non-surgical and non-pharmaceutical. This means that patients can avoid the potential side effects and risks associated with medications and surgery. Additionally, chiropractic care is a relatively low-risk treatment option, making it an attractive option for those who may be hesitant to undergo more invasive medical procedures.

Chiropractic care is effective for a wide range of pain conditions, including back pain, neck pain, and headaches. Chiropractors use a variety of techniques and treatments to relieve pain, including spinal adjustments, massage therapy, and other manual therapies. Chiropractors may also use complementary therapies such as nutritional counseling and exercise to help patients manage pain and improve their overall health.

Studies have shown that chiropractic care is an effective treatment for many pain conditions. A 2017 review of research on chiropractic care for low back pain found that chiropractic care was effective in reducing pain and improving function in patients with low back pain. Another study found that chiropractic care was effective in reducing pain and improving function in patients with neck pain.

Chiropractic care is also effective in treating headaches. A 2011 study found that chiropractic care was effective in reducing the frequency and intensity of headaches in patients with migraine headaches. Another study found that chiropractic care was effective in reducing the frequency and intensity of tension headaches.

In addition to being effective in treating pain conditions, chiropractic care is also an effective treatment option for patients with chronic pain. Chronic pain is a complex condition that can be difficult to treat with traditional medical approaches. Chiropractic care offers a non-invasive, drug-free approach to managing chronic pain, making it an attractive option for patients who are looking for alternative treatment options.

Chiropractic care is also effective in improving the overall health of patients. Chiropractors work to improve the function of the spine and other joints, which can help to improve the overall health of the body. Chiropractic care may also be used to help patients manage other health conditions, such as asthma, allergies, and digestive disorders.

Understanding chronic pain

Chronic pain is a complex and often debilitating condition that affects millions of people worldwide. Unlike acute pain, which is usually short-lived and can be traced to a specific injury or illness, chronic pain persists over time and is often difficult to diagnose and treat. It can have a significant impact on a person's physical and emotional well-being, as well as their ability to work, socialize, and enjoy life. Below we will explore the nature of chronic pain, its causes and symptoms, and some of the treatment options available to those who suffer from it.

What is Chronic Pain?

Chronic pain is defined as pain that persists for more than three to six months. It can be caused by a variety of factors, including injury, illness, or a pre-existing condition such as arthritis or fibromyalgia. Unlike acute pain, which serves as a warning signal that something is wrong, chronic pain can continue even after the underlying problem has been resolved. It can be felt in a variety of ways, including burning, stabbing, or aching sensations, and can occur in any part of the body.

Causes and Symptoms of Chronic Pain

Chronic pain can be caused by a variety of factors, including injury, illness, or a pre-existing condition such as arthritis or fibromyalgia. It can also be caused by psychological factors such as stress, anxiety, or depression. In some cases, the cause of chronic pain may be unknown, making it difficult to diagnose and treat.

The symptoms of chronic pain can vary depending on the underlying cause and the part of the body that is affected. Some common symptoms of chronic pain include:

Aching or stiffness in the affected area

Burning or shooting pain

Fatigue or lack of energy

Difficulty sleeping or staying asleep

Mood changes, such as irritability or depression

Reduced mobility or difficulty with physical activities

Treatment Options for Chronic Pain

Treatment for chronic pain can vary depending on the underlying cause and the severity of the symptoms. In some cases, pain medication may be prescribed to help manage the symptoms of chronic pain. However, medication alone may not be enough to provide long-term relief, and can be associated with side effects and risks.

Chiropractic care is a non-invasive, drug-free approach to managing chronic pain that focuses on the body's natural ability to heal itself. Chiropractors use a variety of techniques, including spinal manipulation, massage therapy, and other manual therapies, to help relieve pain, improve mobility, and restore function.

Spinal manipulation, also known as chiropractic adjustment, is a common technique used by chiropractors to relieve pain and improve function. During a spinal manipulation, the chiropractor applies a controlled force to the joints of the spine, with the goal of improving alignment and reducing pain.

Massage therapy is another common technique used by chiropractors to relieve pain and improve function. Massage therapy involves the manipulation of soft tissues, including muscles and connective tissues, to improve circulation, reduce tension, and promote relaxation.

Other manual therapies used by chiropractors to manage chronic pain include trigger point therapy, which involves applying pressure to specific points on the body to relieve pain, and myofascial release, which involves stretching and releasing the connective tissues that surround muscles.

In addition to these manual therapies, chiropractors may also recommend lifestyle changes to help manage chronic pain. This can include exercise and stretching programs, dietary changes, and stress management techniques such as meditation or relaxation exercises.

Alternative to pain medications

Chronic pain affects millions of people worldwide and is one of the leading causes of disability. While pain medications are commonly used to manage pain, they often come with unwanted side effects and can be addictive. As a result, many people are seeking alternative forms of pain management. Chiropractic care is a non-invasive, drug-free approach to pain management that has been shown to be effective for a wide range of conditions. Below we will explore the role of chiropractic in pain management and how it provides an alternative to pain medications.

Chiropractic is a form of healthcare that focuses on the musculoskeletal system and nervous system. It involves the diagnosis and treatment of mechanical disorders of the musculoskeletal system, especially the spine. Chiropractic care is based on the principle that the body has the ability to heal itself, and that proper alignment of the musculoskeletal system is essential for good health.

Chiropractic care is often used to manage pain caused by conditions such as back pain, neck pain, headaches, and joint pain. Chiropractors use a variety of techniques to help alleviate pain and improve function, including spinal manipulation, mobilization, and soft tissue therapy.

One of the benefits of chiropractic care is that it is non-invasive and drug-free. Pain medications, on the other hand, can be highly addictive and come with a range of side effects, such as nausea, dizziness, and constipation. In addition, long-term use of pain medications can lead to tolerance, dependence, and addiction.

Chiropractic care is also a cost-effective approach to pain management. A study published in the Journal of Manipulative and Physiological Therapeutics found that chiropractic care was more cost-effective than medical care for treating low back pain. The study also found that chiropractic care resulted in fewer hospitalizations and surgeries compared to medical care.

Chiropractic care has been shown to be effective for a wide range of conditions that cause pain. For example, a study published in the Journal of the American Medical Association found that chiropractic care was effective for treating chronic low back pain. The study found that chiropractic care was more effective than medication for improving function and reducing pain.

Another study published in the Annals of Internal Medicine found that chiropractic care was effective for treating neck pain. The study found that chiropractic care was more effective than medication for reducing pain and improving function.

Chiropractic care is also effective for treating headaches. A study published in the Journal of Manipulative and Physiological Therapeutics found that chiropractic care was effective for treating tension headaches and migraines. The study found that chiropractic care was more effective than medication for reducing the frequency and intensity of headaches.

Chiropractic care is often used in conjunction with other forms of pain management, such as physical therapy and massage therapy. This multidisciplinary approach can be highly effective for managing pain and improving function.

In addition to providing an alternative to pain medications, chiropractic care also helps address the underlying cause of pain. Pain is often the result of poor alignment or dysfunction in the musculoskeletal system. Chiropractic care helps restore proper alignment and function, which helps alleviate pain and improve overall health.

Chiropractors also provide education and guidance on lifestyle changes that can help reduce pain and improve function. This may include exercise and stretching, ergonomics, and nutrition. By addressing the underlying cause of pain and providing education on self-care, chiropractors help patients achieve long-term pain relief and improved function.

Personalized pain management plans

Pain is a universal experience that affects people of all ages, genders, and backgrounds. The most common approach to managing pain is through the use of medication, which can be effective but also carries risks such as addiction and adverse side effects. For those seeking an alternative to medication, chiropractic care can provide personalized pain management plans that address the root cause of pain and promote overall wellness.

Chiropractic care is a healthcare practice that focuses on the diagnosis and treatment of disorders of the musculoskeletal system, with a particular emphasis on the spine. Chiropractors use hands-on techniques, such as spinal manipulation, to restore proper alignment and function to the body's joints, muscles, and nerves. By doing so, they aim to alleviate pain and promote healing without the use of medication or surgery.

One of the benefits of chiropractic care for pain management is that it provides a personalized approach to treatment. Chiropractors take the time to assess each patient's unique situation and develop a treatment plan tailored to their specific needs. This may involve a combination of chiropractic adjustments, massage therapy, exercise, and lifestyle modifications.

For example, a patient with chronic low back pain may benefit from regular chiropractic adjustments to realign the spine, as well as massage therapy to relieve muscle tension and improve circulation. In addition, their chiropractor may recommend specific exercises to strengthen the muscles supporting the spine and offer guidance on proper posture and ergonomics to prevent future injury.

Chiropractors also work closely with their patients to identify any underlying health conditions or lifestyle factors that may be contributing to their pain. For instance, a patient with chronic migraines may benefit from dietary changes or stress-reduction techniques in addition to chiropractic adjustments.

Another advantage of chiropractic care for pain management is that it can be used as an alternative to medication. While medication can provide temporary relief, it does not address the root cause of pain and can lead to side effects and addiction. Chiropractic care, on the other hand, is a natural and non-invasive approach to pain management that focuses on restoring the body's natural balance and promoting healing.

Research has shown that chiropractic care can be effective in reducing pain for a variety of conditions, including low back pain, neck pain, headaches, and fibromyalgia. A 2018 study published in the Journal of Alternative and Complementary Medicine found that chiropractic care was more effective than medication for treating acute and chronic low back pain. Another study published in the Journal of Manipulative and Physiological

Therapeutics found that chiropractic care was effective in reducing neck pain and improving function.

In addition to being effective, chiropractic care is also safe. Chiropractors undergo extensive training and are licensed healthcare professionals who are trained to recognize when a patient's condition requires further medical attention. Chiropractic adjustments are gentle and non-invasive and are performed only after a thorough assessment of the patient's health and medical history.

Chapter Eighteen

Chiropractic for Seniors

As people age, their bodies undergo a lot of changes, including a decrease in bone density, muscle mass, and flexibility. These changes often result in chronic pain and discomfort, which can significantly affect their quality of life. Chiropractic care is a safe and effective way for seniors to manage their pain and improve their overall health and wellbeing.

Chiropractic care is a non-invasive, drug-free approach to healthcare that focuses on the diagnosis, treatment, and prevention of musculoskeletal disorders. It involves the use of manual techniques such as spinal manipulation, soft tissue mobilization, and stretching to restore joint mobility and alleviate pain. Chiropractors also provide lifestyle advice, nutritional counseling, and exercise programs to help patients achieve optimal health.

The benefits of chiropractic care for seniors are numerous. First and foremost, it can help reduce pain and improve joint mobility. As people age, the wear and tear on their joints can lead to arthritis, which can cause chronic pain and stiffness. Chiropractic care can help alleviate these symptoms by restoring joint mobility and reducing inflammation.

In addition to pain relief, chiropractic care can also help seniors maintain their balance and prevent falls. Falls are a significant health risk for seniors, as they can result in fractures, head injuries, and other serious health problems. Chiropractic care can help improve balance and coordination, which can reduce the risk of falls and improve overall mobility.

Another benefit of chiropractic care for seniors is improved immune function. As people age, their immune system becomes less effective, which can lead to an increased risk of infection and illness. Chiropractic care has been shown to improve immune function by reducing stress and inflammation in the body.

Chiropractic care is also a safe and effective alternative to medication for seniors who suffer from chronic pain. Many seniors are reluctant to take medication due to concerns about side effects and the risk of addiction. Chiropractic care offers a natural and safe way to manage pain without the use of drugs.

Chiropractic care is a holistic approach to healthcare that focuses on treating the whole person, not just their symptoms. Chiropractors work with seniors to identify the underlying causes of their pain and develop personalized treatment plans that address their unique needs and goals. This approach can help seniors achieve better overall health and wellbeing.

When seeking chiropractic care, seniors should look for a practitioner who has experience working with older adults. They should also look for a practitioner who is willing to work with their primary care physician to ensure that all aspects of their healthcare are coordinated.

Age-related spinal changes

As we age, our bodies undergo numerous changes, and the spine is no exception. Age-related spinal changes can result in a range of issues, from discomfort and pain to decreased mobility and function. Chiropractic care can be a valuable tool in addressing these issues and promoting spinal health in seniors.

One of the most common age-related spinal changes is degenerative disc disease. Over time, the discs between the vertebrae can become thinner and less pliable, leading to decreased shock absorption and mobility. This can result in pain, stiffness, and a reduced range of motion. Chiropractic adjustments can help alleviate these symptoms by improving joint mobility and reducing inflammation.

Another common issue in seniors is spinal stenosis, which occurs when the spinal canal narrows and puts pressure on the spinal cord or nerves. This can lead to pain, tingling, numbness, and weakness in the arms and legs. Chiropractic adjustments can help improve spinal alignment and reduce pressure on the nerves, providing relief from these symptoms.

Osteoporosis, a condition that causes the bones to become brittle and weak, is also a concern for many seniors. As the bones in the spine become weaker, they are more susceptible to fractures and other injuries. Chiropractic adjustments can help improve spinal alignment and reduce the risk of these injuries by promoting better posture and balance.

In addition to these age-related spinal changes, seniors may also experience other health conditions that can impact spinal health, such as arthritis, fibromyalgia, and chronic pain. Chiropractic care can be an effective complementary therapy for these conditions, helping to reduce pain and improve overall function.

When providing chiropractic care to seniors, it is important to take into account their unique needs and concerns. Many seniors may have other health issues or limitations that need to be considered when developing a treatment plan. Chiropractors who specialize in senior care can provide individualized care that takes into account these factors and helps promote overall health and wellness.

Benefits for older adults

Chiropractic care is a non-invasive and drug-free approach to treating a variety of health conditions, and it can be particularly beneficial for older adults. As people age, their bodies undergo a number of changes, including degenerative changes in the spine, which can lead to pain, stiffness, and decreased mobility. Chiropractic care can help address these issues and improve overall health and well-being for seniors.

One of the main benefits of chiropractic care for older adults is pain relief. As the body ages, joints, muscles, and bones can become weakened and more prone to injury. This can lead to chronic pain and discomfort, especially in the neck, back, and joints. Chiropractic adjustments can help relieve this pain by correcting spinal misalignments and reducing pressure on nerves and other soft tissues.

Chiropractic care can also improve range of motion and mobility, which can be particularly important for seniors. As people age, they may experience a loss of flexibility and mobility, which can make everyday tasks more difficult and increase the risk of falls and injuries. Chiropractic adjustments and other techniques can help improve joint mobility and flexibility, which can help seniors stay active and independent.

In addition to pain relief and improved mobility, chiropractic care can also have a positive impact on overall health and wellness. Regular chiropractic adjustments can help improve circulation, boost the immune system, and promote better sleep. This can lead to improved energy levels, better mental clarity, and an overall sense of well-being.

Another benefit of chiropractic care for seniors is that it is a non-invasive and drug-free approach to treatment. As people age, they may be taking multiple medications to manage various health conditions, which can lead to a variety of unwanted side effects. Chiropractic care offers a natural and safe alternative to medication, which can help seniors avoid these side effects and improve their overall quality of life.

Chiropractic care is also highly customizable, which means that it can be tailored to meet the specific needs and health concerns of individual seniors. Chiropractors can work with older adults to develop personalized treatment plans that address their unique health concerns and goals. This may include a combination of chiropractic adjustments, exercise and stretching programs, and lifestyle recommendations to promote better health and well-being.

Chiropractic care for specific age-related conditions

As people age, their bodies undergo many changes that can lead to various health conditions. Chiropractic care is a holistic approach to healthcare that aims to improve the function of the nervous and musculoskeletal systems. This can provide numerous benefits for seniors, particularly those with age-related conditions.

One of the most common age-related conditions that chiropractic care can help with is osteoarthritis. This condition affects the joints and can lead to pain, stiffness, and a reduced range of motion. Chiropractic adjustments can help improve joint function and reduce inflammation, which can help alleviate these symptoms.

Another condition that chiropractic care can help with is degenerative disc disease. This condition affects the spinal discs, which can lead to pain and reduced mobility. Chiropractic adjustments can help improve spinal alignment, reduce pressure on the discs, and improve spinal function, which can alleviate these symptoms.

Seniors are also at an increased risk of falling, which can lead to fractures and other injuries. Chiropractic care can help improve balance and co-ordination, which can reduce the risk of falls. Additionally, chiropractic adjustments can help alleviate pain and stiffness that may be contributing to balance and mobility issues.

Chiropractic care can also be beneficial for seniors with chronic pain conditions, such as fibromyalgia. This condition can cause widespread pain, fatigue, and other symptoms. Chiropractic adjustments can help alleviate pain and improve mobility, which can help improve quality of life for seniors with fibromyalgia.

Another benefit of chiropractic care for seniors is improved immune function. As people age, their immune system becomes less effective, which can lead to an increased risk of infections and other health problems. Chiropractic adjustments can help improve nerve function, which can help improve immune system function and reduce the risk of infections and illnesses.

Finally, chiropractic care can help improve overall quality of life for seniors. As people age, they may experience a reduced ability to perform daily tasks and participate in activities they enjoy. Chiropractic care can help improve mobility and reduce pain, which can help seniors maintain their independence and continue to enjoy their hobbies and interests.

Chapter Nineteen

Chiropractic and Mental Health

Chiropractic care is a holistic approach to healthcare that has been gaining popularity for its ability to address a wide range of health conditions. One area in which chiropractic care has shown promise is in the field of mental health. While it is not a replacement for traditional mental health treatments, chiropractic care can be a helpful complement to other therapies.

Chiropractic care is based on the principle that the body has an innate ability to heal itself. The focus of chiropractic care is on the spine, which is believed to be the foundation of the body. The spinal column houses the spinal cord, which is the communication center between the brain and the rest of the body. Any misalignments or subluxations in the spine can interfere with the nervous system's ability to communicate properly, leading to a range of health problems, including mental health issues.

The nervous system is responsible for regulating the body's functions, including the release of hormones and neurotransmitters that affect mood and behavior. Chiropractic care can help to improve nervous system function by correcting spinal misalignments, which can help to reduce stress and promote a sense of calm.

One of the main benefits of chiropractic care for mental health is its ability to reduce stress. Stress is a major contributor to many mental health problems, including anxiety and depression. Chiropractic adjustments can help to reduce stress levels by promoting relaxation and improving the body's ability to cope with stress.

Chiropractic care can also help to improve sleep quality, which is another important factor in mental health. Many people with mental health problems struggle with sleep issues, which can exacerbate their symptoms. Chiropractic adjustments can help to improve sleep quality by reducing pain and tension in the body, which can make it easier to fall asleep and stay asleep.

Another benefit of chiropractic care for mental health is its ability to improve posture. Poor posture can lead to a range of health problems, including back pain, neck pain, and headaches. It can also contribute to feelings of depression and anxiety. Chiropractic care can help to improve posture by realigning the spine, which can help to reduce pain and tension in the body and promote a sense of wellbeing.

Chiropractic care can also be helpful for people with conditions such as ADHD and autism. These conditions are believed to be linked to nervous system dysfunction, and chiropractic care can help to improve nervous system function by correcting spinal misalignments. While chiropractic care is not a cure for these conditions, it can be a helpful complement to other treatments.

It is important to note that chiropractic care is not a replacement for traditional mental health treatments. People with mental health problems should always seek the guidance of a qualified mental health professional. Chiropractic care can be a helpful complement to other therapies, but it is not a standalone treatment for mental health conditions.

The mind-body connection

The mind-body connection is a well-established concept that recognizes the interrelationship between the mind and the body. The mind and body are not separate entities but are instead deeply interconnected. The way we think, feel, and act can have a significant impact on our physical health, and conversely, the state of our physical health can affect our mental and emotional well-being.

Chiropractic care is a form of alternative medicine that is focused on the diagnosis and treatment of musculoskeletal disorders, particularly those related to the spine. While chiropractic is primarily associated with physical health, it has also been shown to have a positive impact on mental health and well-being.

One of the key ways in which chiropractic care can influence mental health is through its effect on the nervous system. The nervous system is responsible for the regulation of all bodily functions, including those related to mental and emotional well-being. When the spine is misaligned, it can cause interference with the nervous system, leading to a variety of physical and emotional symptoms. By realigning the spine and removing interference, chiropractic care can help to restore balance to the nervous system, leading to improved mental health.

Another way in which chiropractic care can impact mental health is through its effect on the body's natural healing processes. When the body is in a state of pain or dysfunction, it can trigger the release of stress hormones such as cortisol. These hormones can have a negative impact on mental health, leading to symptoms such as anxiety and depression. By addressing the underlying cause of pain and dysfunction, chiropractic care can help to reduce stress on the body, leading to a reduction in stress hormones and improved mental health.

Chiropractic care has also been shown to be an effective treatment for conditions such as anxiety and depression. While these conditions are often treated with medication and psychotherapy, chiropractic care offers a non-invasive and drug-free alternative. By addressing the physical symptoms of these conditions, such as tension and pain, chiropractic care can help to alleviate the associated mental and emotional symptoms.

Chiropractic care can also be beneficial for individuals who have experienced trauma or other emotional stressors. Trauma can manifest physically in the body, leading to pain and dysfunction. By addressing these physical symptoms, chiropractic care can help to reduce the impact of trauma on mental health.

In addition to its direct impact on mental health, chiropractic care can also be beneficial for individuals who are undergoing treatment for mental health conditions. For example, individuals who are taking medication for conditions such as depression and anxiety may experience side effects such as muscle tension and pain. Chiropractic care can help to alleviate these symptoms, making it easier for individuals to manage their condition.

Stress reduction and relaxation

Chiropractic care is often associated with treating physical conditions such as back pain and neck pain, but it can also be an effective way to reduce stress and promote relaxation. Stress is a common problem in today's fast-paced society, and it can lead to a wide range of health problems if left untreated. Chiropractic care can help reduce stress and promote relaxation by addressing physical issues that may be contributing to stress and by improving the overall functioning of the nervous system.

Chiropractic care can help reduce stress by addressing physical issues that may be contributing to stress. For example, chronic pain can be a major source of stress, and chiropractic care can help alleviate pain by addressing underlying musculoskeletal problems. Chiropractors use a variety of techniques to correct misalignments and improve joint function, which can help reduce pain and improve mobility. This can lead to a reduction in stress and an improvement in overall quality of life.

In addition to addressing physical issues, chiropractic care can also help promote relaxation by improving the functioning of the nervous system. The nervous system plays a key role in regulating stress and relaxation responses in the body, and any dysfunction in the nervous system can contribute to stress and anxiety. Chiropractors use a variety of techniques to improve nervous system function, including spinal adjustments, massage therapy, and other modalities. By improving nervous system function, chiropractic care can help reduce stress and promote relaxation.

One of the key ways that chiropractic care promotes relaxation is by reducing muscle tension. Chronic muscle tension is a common problem in individuals who are under stress, and it can lead to a wide range of physical problems such as headaches, neck pain, and back pain. Chiropractors can use a variety of techniques to release muscle tension, including manual adjustments, massage therapy, and stretching exercises. By reducing muscle tension, chiropractic care can help promote relaxation and improve overall quality of life.

Chiropractic care can also help reduce stress by promoting better sleep. Chronic stress can interfere with sleep patterns, leading to problems such as insomnia and fatigue. Chiropractors can help address sleep problems by addressing underlying musculoskeletal problems that may be interfering with sleep. For example, misalignments in the spine can cause pain and discomfort that make it difficult to get comfortable at night. By correcting these misalignments, chiropractors can help improve sleep quality and reduce stress levels.

In addition to promoting relaxation and reducing stress, chiropractic care can also help improve mental health. There is a growing body of research that suggests that chiropractic care may be effective in treating conditions such as anxiety and depression. One study published in the Journal of Upper Cervical Chiropractic Research found that chiropractic care can help reduce symptoms of depression in individuals with chronic pain. Another study published in the Journal of Manipulative and Physiological Therapeutics found that chiropractic care can help reduce symptoms of anxiety in individuals with a history of anxiety disorders.

Chiropractic care can also help improve overall wellness by promoting healthy lifestyle habits. Chiropractors often provide patients with advice on nutrition, exercise, and other lifestyle factors that can help reduce stress and improve overall health. For example, chiropractors may recommend a healthy diet that includes plenty of fruits and vegetables, as well as regular exercise to help reduce stress and promote relaxation.

Chiropractic's role in improving mental well-being

Chiropractic care is often associated with treating physical pain and injuries, but it can also have a positive impact on mental well-being. The connection between physical health and mental health is well established, and chiropractic care can play a role in improving both.

One way that chiropractic care can benefit mental well-being is by reducing physical pain. Chronic pain can cause significant psychological distress, including depression, anxiety, and decreased quality of life. Chiropractic adjustments have been shown to be effective in reducing pain in a variety of conditions, including back pain, neck pain, and headaches. By reducing pain levels, chiropractic care can improve a patient's mood, decrease stress levels, and improve overall well-being.

Chiropractic care can also help to reduce stress levels. Stress is a common cause of both physical and mental health problems. It can lead to tension headaches, back pain, and digestive problems, as well as contribute to depression and anxiety. Chiropractic adjustments have been shown to reduce levels of cortisol, the hormone associated with stress, and increase levels of serotonin and dopamine, the hormones associated with happiness and relaxation.

In addition to physical adjustments, chiropractors often provide lifestyle advice and guidance on exercise and nutrition. This holistic approach to health can have a positive impact on mental well-being. For example, regular exercise has been shown to be effective in reducing symptoms of depression and anxiety, and a healthy diet can improve mood and cognitive function.

Another way that chiropractic care can improve mental well-being is by promoting better sleep. Sleep is essential for overall health and well-being, and poor sleep is associated with a range of physical and mental health problems, including depression and anxiety. Chiropractic adjustments have been shown to be effective in improving sleep quality and duration, which can in turn improve mental health.

Chiropractors can also play a role in helping patients manage specific mental health conditions. For example, chiropractic care has been shown to be effective in reducing symptoms of attention deficit hyperactivity disorder (ADHD) in children. Chiropractors can work with other healthcare professionals to develop a comprehensive treatment plan for patients with mental health conditions.

It is important to note that chiropractic care should not be used as a replacement for mental health treatment, such as therapy or medication.

However, it can be an effective complementary treatment option for those looking to improve their overall physical and mental health.

Chapter Twenty

Chiropractic for Animal Care

Chiropractic is a healthcare profession that is primarily focused on the diagnosis, treatment, and prevention of musculoskeletal disorders, particularly those affecting the spine. While chiropractic care is primarily associated with the human body, it can also be utilized to treat animals, including dogs, cats, horses, and other livestock. Chiropractic care for animals is a rapidly growing field that is gaining more attention and recognition among animal owners and veterinarians alike.

The principles of chiropractic care for animals are similar to those used in humans. The goal of chiropractic care is to help the body heal itself by restoring proper spinal alignment and improving the function of the nervous system. When the spine is misaligned, it can lead to a range of health problems, including joint pain, muscle tension, and nerve dysfunction. Chiropractors use manual manipulation techniques to correct these spinal misalignments, known as subluxations.

Animals, like humans, can also suffer from subluxations. However, they are often more difficult to detect and diagnose because animals cannot communicate their symptoms in the same way that humans can. Some of the signs that an animal may be suffering from a subluxation include changes in gait or posture, stiffness, reluctance to move or play, and decreased mobility or flexibility. Chiropractors who specialize in animal care are trained to identify these subtle signs and perform manual adjustments to correct the problem.

One of the benefits of chiropractic care for animals is that it is a non-invasive and drug-free treatment option. Many traditional veterinary treatments rely on medications or surgeries to address health problems. While these treatments can be effective in some cases, they often come with risks and potential side effects. Chiropractic care, on the other hand, uses gentle manipulation techniques to promote natural healing without the need for medication or surgery.

Another benefit of chiropractic care for animals is that it can be used to treat a wide range of conditions. In addition to musculoskeletal disorders, chiropractic care can also be used to address digestive issues, respiratory problems, and even behavioral issues. By improving spinal alignment and nervous system function, chiropractic care can help animals to feel more comfortable and relaxed, which can lead to improvements in overall health and well-being.

Chiropractic care for animals is becoming more widely accepted among veterinary professionals. In fact, many veterinary schools now offer courses in animal chiropractic care, and there are a growing number of chiropractors who specialize in animal care. Additionally, several states have passed laws allowing licensed chiropractors to provide chiropractic care to animals.

When seeking chiropractic care for an animal, it is important to choose a chiropractor who has specialized training and experience in animal care. A chiropractor who works primarily with humans may not be familiar with the unique anatomy and physiology of animals, which can lead to improper treatment and potential harm. It is also important to work closely with a veterinarian to ensure that chiropractic care is an appropriate treatment option for the animal's specific condition.

History and application

Chiropractic is a healthcare profession that has been around for over a century. It is primarily concerned with the diagnosis and treatment of musculoskeletal and nervous system disorders, with a focus on the spine. While chiropractic was originally developed as a human healthcare practice, it has also been adapted for use in animal care.

The history of chiropractic dates back to 1895 when Daniel David Palmer, a magnetic healer, performed the first chiropractic adjustment on a janitor who had a hearing problem. This led to the discovery of the relationship between the spinal column and the nervous system. Palmer believed that misalignments in the spine (known as subluxations) were the root cause of many health problems, and that correcting these misalignments could help restore the body's natural ability to heal itself.

The application of chiropractic in animal care is relatively new, with the first veterinary chiropractic association being established in the United States in 1989. Since then, the practice has gained popularity and acceptance, and there are now many licensed animal chiropractors throughout the world.

The principles of chiropractic in animal care are similar to those in human care. Animal chiropractors focus on detecting and correcting subluxations in the spine and other joints of the body. They use manual adjustments and other techniques to restore proper alignment and function of the musculoskeletal and nervous systems. This can help improve mobility, reduce pain, and enhance overall health and well-being in animals.

Animal chiropractic can be used to treat a variety of conditions, including musculoskeletal injuries, neurological disorders, and chronic pain. It can also be used as a preventative measure to maintain optimal health and performance in animals, particularly in performance animals such as horses and dogs.

One of the benefits of chiropractic in animal care is that it is non-invasive and drug-free. This can be particularly beneficial for animals that may be sensitive or allergic to medications. Chiropractic can also be used in conjunction with other veterinary treatments to enhance their effectiveness.

Animal chiropractors undergo extensive training and education, which includes the study of animal anatomy and physiology, as well as the principles and techniques of chiropractic. They also learn how to perform thorough physical examinations, diagnose conditions, and develop treatment plans.

It is important to note that animal chiropractic should only be performed by a licensed and trained professional. The safety and well-being of the animal should always be the top priority, and the chiropractor should work closely with the animal's primary veterinarian to ensure that the best possible care is provided.

Benefits for animals

Chiropractic care is not just for humans, but it can also be beneficial for animals. Chiropractic for animal care is a growing field that focuses on the detection and correction of spinal and joint dysfunctions in animals. It is based on the same principles and techniques as chiropractic care for humans, but adapted to suit the anatomy and physiology of animals.

The application of chiropractic care for animal care has a long history, with evidence of spinal manipulation being used to treat animal injuries dating back to ancient civilizations. In modern times, veterinary chiropractic care has become more mainstream, with many veterinarians and animal chiropractors offering chiropractic care for animals.

Chiropractic care for animals can benefit them in many ways. One of the primary benefits is pain relief. Animals, just like humans, can suffer from musculoskeletal injuries, and chiropractic care can help to alleviate pain and discomfort caused by these injuries. Additionally, chiropractic care can improve mobility and flexibility in animals, which can be especially important for older animals or those with chronic conditions that affect their mobility.

Chiropractic care can also improve overall health and well-being in animals. By correcting spinal and joint dysfunctions, chiropractic care can help to restore proper nerve function and blood flow to various parts of the body, which can improve organ function and overall health. Additionally, chiropractic care can help to prevent injuries and promote a faster recovery from injuries.

There are many different types of animals that can benefit from chiropractic care. Some of the most common animals that receive chiropractic care include dogs, cats, horses, and other large animals such as cows and sheep. Chiropractic care can also be beneficial for animals used in sports and competitions, such as racehorses, agility dogs, and show animals.

When it comes to chiropractic care for animals, it is important to work with a trained and licensed animal chiropractor. Animal chiropractors are trained to work with animals and understand the differences in anatomy and physiology between different species. They can perform chiropractic adjustments on animals safely and effectively, using techniques that are appropriate for the specific animal being treated.

In addition to chiropractic adjustments, animal chiropractors may also recommend other therapies or treatments to help support the animal's health and well-being. This may include massage, acupuncture, and nutritional counseling, among other things.

It is also important to note that chiropractic care should not be used as a replacement for traditional veterinary care. Animal chiropractors work in conjunction with veterinarians to provide a comprehensive treatment plan for the animal. Chiropractic care is just one part of a larger plan to support the animal's health and well-being.

Techniques for various species

Chiropractic care is not limited to humans, and can be applied to a variety of animal species as well. Just like in humans, the goal of chiropractic care for animals is to improve the function of the musculoskeletal system, thereby enhancing overall health and wellbeing. Chiropractic care for animals has been gaining popularity in recent years, with many veterinarians and animal owners recognizing the benefits of this alternative approach to animal care.

There are various techniques that can be used for chiropractic care in animals. One of the most commonly used techniques is the diversified technique, which involves the use of high-velocity, low-amplitude thrusts to adjust misaligned joints. This technique is often used for larger animals, such as horses and cows. Another commonly used technique is the activator method, which involves the use of a handheld instrument to deliver a low-force adjustment. This technique is often used for smaller animals, such as dogs and cats.

Chiropractic care can be beneficial for a variety of animal species, including horses, dogs, cats, and even exotic animals like birds and reptiles. In horses, chiropractic care can be used to address issues such as lameness, back pain, and poor performance. Regular chiropractic care can help to improve joint mobility, reduce muscle tension, and promote overall balance and coordination.

In dogs and cats, chiropractic care can be used to address issues such as arthritis, hip dysplasia, and other musculoskeletal conditions. Chiropractic adjustments can help to reduce pain and inflammation, improve range of motion, and enhance overall mobility. Chiropractic care can also be used to address issues related to behavior, such as anxiety and aggression. By improving overall comfort and wellbeing, chiropractic care can help to improve a pet's behavior and reduce stress.

Chiropractic care can also be used for exotic animals, such as birds and reptiles. In these animals, chiropractic care can be used to address issues such as wing or leg paralysis, spinal misalignments, and other musculoskeletal conditions. Chiropractic adjustments can help to improve mobility and reduce pain, thereby enhancing overall quality of life.

In addition to the physical benefits of chiropractic care for animals, there are also emotional benefits. Chiropractic care is a non-invasive approach to animal care, which can help to reduce stress and anxiety. Many animals find chiropractic adjustments to be relaxing and soothing, which can help to promote a sense of calm and wellbeing.

It is important to note that chiropractic care for animals should always be performed by a licensed and experienced animal chiropractor. Animal chiropractors are trained to understand the unique anatomy and physiology of different animal species, and can tailor their techniques and approach to meet the specific needs of each individual animal.

Chapter Twenty-One

Chiropractic Education and Training

Chiropractic is a healthcare profession that is dedicated to the diagnosis and treatment of musculoskeletal disorders, primarily the spine. It focuses on the relationship between the body's structure, primarily the spine, and its function, as well as the role of the nervous system in health and disease. Chiropractic treatment includes manual adjustments or manipulations of the spine, as well as other therapeutic interventions.

To become a chiropractor, individuals must undergo extensive education and training. The education and training required to become a chiropractor can vary from country to country, but most countries require a minimum of three years of undergraduate education and an additional four years of chiropractic education. In addition, most countries require that chiropractors pass a licensing exam before they can practice.

Chiropractic education programs typically consist of a combination of classroom instruction, laboratory work, and clinical experience. Coursework covers a range of topics including anatomy, physiology, pathology, chiropractic philosophy and principles, diagnosis, and treatment. Students also receive extensive training in manual manipulation techniques, as well as other therapeutic interventions such as therapeutic exercise, nutrition, and patient counseling.

One of the hallmarks of chiropractic education is the emphasis on hands-on training. Students receive extensive instruction in manual manipulation techniques, which are a core component of chiropractic treatment. This hands-on training helps students develop the skills and expertise needed to safely and effectively treat patients with musculoskeletal disorders.

Chiropractic education also emphasizes the importance of evidence-based practice. Students learn how to critically evaluate scientific research, and how to apply that research to their clinical practice. This focus on evidence-based practice helps ensure that chiropractors are providing the most effective and safest care possible to their patients.

In addition to the education and training required to become a chiropractor, many chiropractors also pursue additional education and training in specialized areas of practice. For example, some chiropractors may choose to specialize in sports chiropractic, pediatric chiropractic, or chiropractic neurology. These specialized areas of practice require additional education and training beyond what is typically required to become a chiropractor.

Continuing education is also an important part of chiropractic practice. Chiropractors are required to complete a certain number of continuing education hours each year to maintain their licensure. This continuing education helps chiropractors stay up-to-date on the latest research and treatment techniques, and ensures that they are providing the highest quality of care to their patients.

Chiropractic education and training are constantly evolving to keep pace with the latest research and developments in the field. As our understanding of the musculoskeletal system and the role of the nervous system in health and disease continues to advance, so too does chiropractic education and training.

In recent years, there has been a growing recognition of the importance of interprofessional collaboration in healthcare. Chiropractors are increasingly working alongside other healthcare professionals such as medical doctors, physical therapists, and massage therapists to provide patients with comprehensive, integrated care.

Chiropractic colleges and programs

Chiropractic is a form of alternative medicine that focuses on the diagnosis and treatment of musculoskeletal disorders, particularly spinal disorders. It is a non-invasive, hands-on approach to healthcare that uses spinal manipulation and other manual therapies to improve the body's alignment and function. To become a licensed chiropractor, an individual must undergo extensive education and training in this field.

Chiropractic education typically begins with a bachelor's degree in a related field, such as biology, chemistry, or anatomy. After completing an undergraduate degree, individuals interested in pursuing a career in chiropractic must enroll in a chiropractic college or program. There are over 20 accredited chiropractic programs in the United States, and each program has specific admission requirements.

Chiropractic programs typically take four years to complete and include both classroom and clinical training. In the first two years of the program, students take courses in anatomy, physiology, pathology, microbiology, biochemistry, and other basic sciences. During the second two years, students receive extensive clinical training in chiropractic techniques, patient assessment, diagnosis, and treatment.

The clinical training component of chiropractic education is an essential part of the curriculum. It provides students with the opportunity to apply the knowledge and skills they have learned in the classroom to real patients. Under the supervision of licensed chiropractors, students learn to perform spinal manipulation and other manual therapies, as well as develop treatment plans and communicate with patients.

In addition to completing a chiropractic program, individuals must also pass a national board exam to become licensed to practice chiropractic in their state. The National Board of Chiropractic Examiners (NBCE) administers the exam, which assesses a candidate's knowledge and clinical skills in various areas, including chiropractic techniques, diagnostic imaging, and patient management.

Continuing education is also an important aspect of a chiropractor's training. To maintain their license, chiropractors must participate in ongoing education and training throughout their career. Continuing education courses can include advanced chiropractic techniques, new research developments, and other related topics.

Chiropractic education and training are designed to provide students with a solid foundation in the principles and practices of chiropractic medicine. Graduates of chiropractic programs are equipped with the knowledge and skills necessary to diagnose and treat musculoskeletal disorders using manual therapies and other non-invasive techniques. They also have the ability to communicate effectively with patients, collaborate with other healthcare providers, and provide preventative care and wellness advice.

In recent years, there has been an increasing demand for chiropractic services. This has led to a growing number of chiropractic programs and an expansion of chiropractic services in various healthcare settings, including hospitals, clinics, and private practices. As a result, there are many opportunities for individuals interested in pursuing a career in chiropractic.

Coursework and clinical experience

Chiropractic is a healthcare profession that focuses on diagnosing and treating conditions related to the musculoskeletal system. The musculoskeletal system includes the bones, joints, muscles, tendons, and ligaments. Chiropractic care involves the use of manual manipulation and other therapies to relieve pain, improve function, and promote overall health and wellness. Chiropractors undergo rigorous education and training to become licensed professionals.

To become a chiropractor, one must complete a Doctor of Chiropractic (DC) degree program at an accredited chiropractic college. These programs typically take four years to complete and require a minimum of three years of undergraduate education. Admission requirements vary by school, but most programs require a minimum GPA and completion of prerequisite courses in biology, chemistry, and other sciences.

The coursework in chiropractic programs covers a wide range of topics related to human anatomy, physiology, and biomechanics, as well as diagnosis and treatment of musculoskeletal conditions. Some common courses in chiropractic programs include anatomy and physiology, pathology, neurology, radiology, and chiropractic technique. Students also receive hands-on clinical experience under the supervision of licensed chiropractors.

In addition to the core curriculum, many chiropractic programs offer elective courses and specialized training in areas such as sports chiropractic, pediatric chiropractic, and nutrition. Some chiropractors choose to pursue postgraduate education and training in these areas to further their expertise and provide more specialized care to their patients.

Upon completion of a chiropractic program, graduates must pass national and state licensing exams to become licensed chiropractors. Licensing requirements vary by state, but typically include completion of an accredited chiropractic program and passing the National Board of Chiropractic Examiners (NBCE) exams. Chiropractors must also meet ongoing continuing education requirements to maintain their licensure and stay up to date on the latest advances in their field.

The clinical experience component of chiropractic education is an essential part of the training process. Chiropractic students typically begin their clinical experience in their third year of study, working in campus clinics and under the supervision of licensed chiropractors. In their fourth year, students typically complete an off-campus clinical internship, where they gain experience working in a variety of healthcare settings and treating patients with a wide range of musculoskeletal conditions.

The clinical experience component of chiropractic education is an essential part of the training process. Chiropractic students typically begin their clinical experience in their third year of study, working in campus clinics and under the supervision of licensed chiropractors. In their fourth year, students typically complete an off-campus clinical internship, where they gain experience working in a variety of healthcare settings and treating patients with a wide range of musculoskeletal conditions.

Chiropractic education and training emphasize the importance of evidence-based practice and a patient-centered approach to care. Chiropractors are trained to take a holistic approach to treating their patients, considering the whole person and not just the specific condition or symptoms they present with. This includes taking into account the patient's lifestyle, diet, and overall health when developing treatment plans.

Board examinations and certification

Chiropractic is a healthcare profession that focuses on the diagnosis, treatment, and prevention of disorders related to the musculoskeletal system and the nervous system. Chiropractors employ various techniques to adjust and manipulate the spine and other joints in the body to alleviate pain and restore proper function. To become a licensed chiropractor, one must undergo extensive education and training, pass board examinations, and obtain certification. Below we will explore the process of becoming a chiropractor and the requirements for board certification.

Chiropractic education typically requires completion of a four-year doctoral program at a chiropractic college accredited by the Council on Chiropractic Education (CCE). The coursework includes foundational courses in anatomy, physiology, biochemistry, microbiology, pathology, and radiology. Additionally, chiropractic students receive extensive training in chiropractic principles, techniques, and clinical practice.

One of the most significant components of chiropractic education is clinical experience. Chiropractic students are required to complete a minimum of 1,000 hours of supervised clinical experience to graduate. During this time, they work with patients under the guidance of licensed chiropractors to develop their skills in diagnosis, treatment planning, and patient management.

1. After graduating from a chiropractic program, aspiring chiropractors must pass a series of board examinations to obtain licensure. The National Board of Chiropractic Examiners (NBCE) administers four exams, including Part I: Basic Science, Part II: Clinical Science, Part III: Clinical Case Management, and Part IV: Practical Examination. Each exam assesses a candidate's knowledge and skills in different areas of chiropractic practice.

In addition to passing the board examinations, chiropractors must obtain licensure from their state's chiropractic licensing board. Requirements for licensure vary by state but typically include completion of a doctoral program, passing the board examinations, and meeting any state-specific requirements.

Board certification is an optional credential that recognizes chiropractors who have demonstrated advanced knowledge and skills in a particular area of practice. The American Board of Chiropractic Specialties (ABCS) offers certification in several areas, including sports chiropractic, chiropractic acupuncture, chiropractic rehabilitation, and chiropractic neurology. To become board certified, chiropractors must complete additional education and training in their chosen specialty and pass an examination.

Board certification is a rigorous process that requires chiropractors to demonstrate expertise in their chosen area of practice. It provides a way for patients and healthcare professionals to identify chiropractors who have gone above and beyond the minimum requirements for licensure and who have demonstrated a commitment to continuing education and professional development.

Chapter Twenty-Two

Chiropractic Practice Management

Chiropractic is a healthcare profession that focuses on the diagnosis and treatment of musculoskeletal disorders, particularly those affecting the spine. Chiropractors are trained to use various manual therapies, such as spinal manipulation and mobilization, to alleviate pain and improve the function of the body. However, chiropractic practice is not limited to patient care alone. Like any other healthcare profession, it also requires effective practice management to ensure that patients receive high-quality care and the practice operates efficiently.

Effective chiropractic practice management involves various aspects such as financial management, staff management, marketing, and communication with patients. Chiropractors must understand and implement these aspects to ensure their practice runs smoothly and effectively.

One essential aspect of practice management is financial management. Chiropractors must keep track of their income and expenses, including billing, insurance claims, and patient records. Proper financial management ensures that the practice remains profitable and financially viable. Chiropractors should regularly analyze their practice's financial performance and make necessary adjustments to improve their revenue streams.

Staff management is also a crucial aspect of practice management. Chiropractors must recruit, train, and retain competent and dedicated staff. The staff must work together to ensure that patients receive optimal care and that the practice operates efficiently. The chiropractor should create a positive work environment that fosters teamwork and collaboration among staff members.

Marketing is another essential aspect of practice management. Chiropractors must promote their practice to attract new patients and retain existing ones. They should develop a strong brand identity and reputation in their community. Effective marketing strategies include developing a website, social media marketing, and engaging in community events.

Communication with patients is vital for successful chiropractic practice management. Chiropractors must establish an effective communication system to engage and educate patients. Effective communication enhances the patient's understanding of their condition and treatment options, resulting in better patient outcomes. Chiropractors should encourage patients to ask questions and provide them with the necessary information to make informed decisions about their health.

Chiropractic practice management also involves ensuring the proper documentation and compliance with regulatory bodies. Chiropractors must maintain accurate records of patient visits, treatments, and billing. They must also comply with state and federal regulations governing the practice of chiropractic.

To ensure effective chiropractic practice management, chiropractors should seek professional development opportunities. Continuing education programs provide chiropractors with up-to-date information on industry trends and best practices. Chiropractors can also benefit from mentorship and networking opportunities within their professional associations.

Establishing a practice

Chiropractic is a healthcare profession that focuses on the diagnosis, treatment, and prevention of disorders related to the musculoskeletal system, particularly the spine. Chiropractors employ various techniques to manipulate or adjust the spine, joints, and muscles to alleviate pain and improve overall bodily function. With the growing demand for alternative therapies, chiropractic has become an attractive field for healthcare professionals looking to establish a practice. Below we will explore the essential steps required to establish a chiropractic practice successfully.

The first step in establishing a chiropractic practice is to obtain the necessary education and training. Aspiring chiropractors must complete a rigorous educational program consisting of a four-year doctoral degree program in chiropractic from an accredited college or university. In addition to coursework in anatomy, physiology, and biomechanics, students are required to complete extensive clinical training in chiropractic techniques, patient management, and diagnosis. After completing their education, prospective chiropractors must pass a national board exam and obtain a state license to practice.

Once licensed, chiropractors can either start their own practice or join an existing practice. Those interested in starting their own practice must consider various factors, including the location, equipment, and staffing requirements. One of the most critical decisions to make when starting a chiropractic practice is choosing the right location. It is essential to choose a location that is accessible to patients and has sufficient space to accommodate the necessary equipment and staff.

Another crucial aspect of establishing a chiropractic practice is purchasing the necessary equipment. Chiropractors require specialized equipment such as chiropractic tables, adjusting tools, and x-ray machines. Investing in high-quality equipment can ensure that patients receive the best possible care while also improving the efficiency and productivity of the practice.

Chiropractors must also consider staffing requirements when establishing a practice. Depending on the size of the practice, chiropractors may need to hire administrative staff, licensed massage therapists, or other healthcare professionals to support patient care. It is essential to hire qualified and dedicated staff who share the chiropractor's vision and commitment to patient care.

Marketing and promotion are also essential components of establishing a successful chiropractic practice. Chiropractors must establish a strong online presence through a website and social media platforms. A website should include information about the practice, including location, services offered, hours of operation, and contact information. Social media platforms can be used to engage with patients, share educational content, and promote the practice.

In addition to online marketing, chiropractors can promote their practice through traditional marketing methods such as direct mail, flyers, and community outreach. Participating in community events, offering free consultations, and partnering with local businesses can help build awareness and attract new patients.

Finally, maintaining a successful chiropractic practice requires ongoing education and training. Chiropractors must stay up-to-date on the latest techniques, research, and regulations to provide the best possible care to their patients. Continuing education programs, seminars, and workshops can provide valuable opportunities for professional growth and development.

Marketing and patient retention

Marketing and patient retention are critical elements in running a successful chiropractic practice. As with any business, marketing is essential for attracting new patients, while patient retention is essential for building and maintaining a strong patient base. Below we will discuss some of the effective marketing and patient retention strategies that chiropractors can use to grow their practices.

Marketing Strategies:

1. Referral marketing: One of the most effective marketing strategies for chiropractors is referral marketing. Referral marketing involves encouraging current patients to refer their friends and family to the practice. To make referral marketing work, the chiropractor needs to ensure that their current patients are satisfied with their services. This can be achieved by providing excellent customer service and quality care.

2. Online marketing: In today's digital age, online marketing is critical for any business. Chiropractors can leverage online marketing strategies to reach out to potential patients. This can include building a professional website that provides information about the practice, creating social media pages, and creating online advertisements.

3. Community outreach: Another effective marketing strategy is community outreach. This involves reaching out to local community organizations and participating in events such as health fairs and charity events. This allows chiropractors to meet potential patients face to face and promote their practice.

Patient Retention Strategies:

4. Quality of care: The primary factor in patient retention is the quality of care provided. Patients will continue to visit a chiropractor who provides quality care that meets their needs. Chiropractors should focus on providing personalized care that addresses the patient's specific needs and concerns.

5. Communication: Good communication is essential for patient retention. Chiropractors should communicate effectively with their patients to ensure that they understand their treatment plan and feel comfortable asking questions. This can be achieved through regular follow-up calls, emails, or in-person appointments.

6. Patient education: Chiropractors should educate their patients about the benefits of chiropractic care and how it can help improve their health and well-being. This can be achieved through educational materials, seminars, and workshops.

7. Convenience: Patients appreciate convenience, and chiropractors can improve patient retention by offering convenient scheduling options, such as online booking, same-day appointments, and extended hours.

Legal and financial considerations

Chiropractic care is a growing field with a lot of potential for success. However, with any business or healthcare practice, there are legal and financial considerations that must be addressed to ensure long-term success. Below we will explore some of the legal and financial considerations that chiropractors must keep in mind when establishing and running a practice.

One of the most important legal considerations for chiropractors is licensing and regulatory compliance. To practice chiropractic, chiropractors must obtain a license from the state in which they plan to practice. Each state has its own licensing board and specific requirements for licensure. In addition, chiropractors must comply with various regulations and guidelines set forth by state and federal agencies. These regulations cover a wide range of areas, including billing and coding practices, patient record keeping, and patient privacy rights.

Another important legal consideration is malpractice insurance. Malpractice insurance protects chiropractors from financial loss in the event of a malpractice lawsuit. The cost of malpractice insurance varies depending on factors such as the location of the practice, the chiropractor's experience, and the scope of services offered. Chiropractors should research and compare different malpractice insurance policies to find one that offers the right amount of coverage at an affordable cost.

In addition to legal considerations, chiropractors must also keep in mind the financial aspects of running a practice. One of the most significant financial considerations is start-up costs. Starting a chiropractic practice requires a significant investment in equipment, office space, and marketing. Chiropractors should create a detailed business plan and budget to determine the necessary start-up costs and secure the necessary funding.

Once the practice is up and running, chiropractors must also consider ongoing expenses such as rent, utilities, and employee salaries. Chiropractors should regularly review their financial statements to ensure that revenue is covering expenses and that the practice is profitable. It is also important to have a financial plan in place for unexpected expenses, such as equipment repairs or legal fees.

Marketing is another crucial aspect of running a successful chiropractic practice. Chiropractors must develop a marketing strategy that effectively promotes their services to potential patients. This can include a variety of tactics, such as online advertising, direct mail campaigns, and community outreach events. Chiropractors should also consider partnering with other healthcare professionals and building relationships with local businesses to increase their visibility and reputation in the community.

In addition to marketing, patient retention is also essential for the long-term success of a chiropractic practice. Chiropractors should focus on building strong relationships with their patients and providing excellent care to encourage patient loyalty. This can include offering flexible scheduling options, providing educational resources on chiropractic care, and incorporating patient feedback into practice improvements.

Finally, it is important for chiropractors to stay up to date on changes and developments in the field. This includes staying informed about new techniques and technologies, attending industry conferences and continuing education courses, and networking with other chiropractors and healthcare professionals. By staying informed and engaged, chiropractors can ensure that they are providing the best possible care to their patients and staying competitive in the market.

Chapter Twenty-Three

Chiropractic Around the World

Chiropractic is a healthcare profession that is growing in popularity and recognition around the world. It focuses on the diagnosis and treatment of neuromusculoskeletal disorders, with an emphasis on spinal manipulation therapy. While chiropractic has its roots in the United States, it has spread to countries all over the world, and each country has its own unique history and approach to the practice.

Canada was one of the first countries outside the United States to embrace chiropractic. The first chiropractic college outside of the US was established in Canada in 1906, and the profession has been regulated and recognized by the government since the 1950s. Today, there are more than 10,000 licensed chiropractors in Canada, and the profession is covered by most private insurance plans and the public healthcare system.

In Europe, chiropractic has a more recent history. The first chiropractic clinic in Europe was established in London in 1924, but the profession did not gain official recognition in most European countries until the late 20th century. Today, there are chiropractors practicing in most European countries, and the profession is regulated by national laws and professional associations.

In Australia, chiropractic has been regulated and recognized since the 1970s, and there are now more than 5,000 licensed chiropractors in the country. Chiropractic is covered by private health insurance, and some chiropractors are also contracted by the government to provide services in public hospitals and clinics.

In Asia, chiropractic is a relatively new profession, with the first chiropractic college in the region opening in Japan in the 1970s. Today, there are chiropractors practicing in many Asian countries, including China, South Korea, and Singapore. However, the profession is not yet widely recognized or regulated in some countries, and there is still some skepticism and misunderstanding about chiropractic among the general public.

In Latin America, chiropractic has been practiced since the early 20th century, but it is only in recent years that the profession has become more widely recognized and regulated by governments. Today, there are chiropractors practicing in most Latin American countries, and the profession is growing in popularity as more people seek alternative healthcare options.

One of the biggest challenges facing chiropractors around the world is the lack of standardization in education and regulation. While many countries have established educational requirements and professional associations, there is still a great deal of variation in the scope of practice and regulatory standards from country to country. This can make it difficult for chiropractors to practice in different countries or to have their qualifications recognized internationally.

Despite these challenges, chiropractic continues to grow and evolve as a healthcare profession around the world. As more people seek out alternative healthcare options and governments recognize the value of non-invasive and drug-free treatments, chiropractic is likely to become an increasingly important part of the global healthcare landscape.

International scope of chiropractic

Chiropractic is a healthcare profession that focuses on the diagnosis, treatment, and prevention of disorders of the musculoskeletal system and the nervous system, and the effects of these disorders on general health. It is a well-established profession in the United States and Canada, but it is also practiced in many other parts of the world. Below we will explore the international scope of chiropractic and its global presence.

The origins of chiropractic can be traced back to the United States in the late 19th century, but it has since spread to other countries around the world. The practice of chiropractic is now recognized and regulated in many countries, including Australia, Canada, Japan, the United Kingdom, and many European countries. In fact, the World Federation of Chiropractic estimates that there are over 100,000 chiropractors practicing in over 90 countries worldwide.

The practice of chiropractic has evolved differently in different parts of the world. For example, in Australia and Canada, chiropractors are primary healthcare providers, meaning that patients can seek chiropractic care without a referral from a medical doctor. In the United Kingdom, however, chiropractors are considered complementary and alternative medicine (CAM) practitioners and work in conjunction with medical doctors and other healthcare professionals. In Japan, chiropractic is not recognized as a separate healthcare profession, but chiropractors are licensed to practice spinal manipulation as part of their physical therapy training.

Despite these differences, chiropractic care generally focuses on the diagnosis and treatment of musculoskeletal conditions, such as back pain, neck pain, and headaches. Chiropractors use a variety of manual techniques, including spinal manipulation and mobilization, to restore joint mobility, reduce pain, and improve function. They also provide advice on lifestyle changes, such as exercise and nutrition, to help patients achieve optimal health.

One area in which chiropractic has gained particular attention is in the management of musculoskeletal conditions in athletes. Chiropractic care is often used in sports medicine to help prevent injuries, improve performance, and speed up recovery from injuries. Many professional sports teams have chiropractors on staff to provide care for their athletes.

Another area in which chiropractic has gained recognition is in the management of chronic pain. Chiropractic care can be an effective non-pharmacological option for managing chronic pain conditions, such as low back pain, neck pain, and fibromyalgia. In some countries, chiropractors work alongside medical doctors to provide a comprehensive approach to pain management.

Despite the growing recognition of chiropractic around the world, there are still some challenges that the profession faces. One of the main challenges is the lack of uniform regulation and licensure standards across different countries. This can make it difficult for chiropractors to practice internationally and for patients to know what kind of care they can expect when seeking chiropractic care in a foreign country.

Another challenge is the lack of research on the effectiveness and safety of chiropractic care, especially in comparison to other treatments for musculoskeletal conditions. While there is some evidence to support the use of chiropractic care for certain conditions, such as low back pain, more research is needed to better understand the benefits and limitations of this treatment approach.

Chiropractic in various cultures

Chiropractic is a healthcare profession that has gained popularity in many cultures around the world. Although it is most commonly associated with Western cultures, chiropractic has been embraced by people from all walks of life and all parts of the globe. Below we will explore the various cultural perspectives of chiropractic and how it has been integrated into different societies.

Chiropractic is rooted in the philosophy that the body has the innate ability to heal itself. It is based on the idea that the nervous system controls every aspect of the body, and that misalignments of the spine can interfere with the nervous system's ability to function properly. By manually adjusting the spine to correct these misalignments, chiropractors aim to restore the body's natural ability to heal itself.

In the United States, chiropractic has been a popular healthcare choice for many years. According to the National Center for Complementary and Integrative Health, chiropractic is one of the most commonly used complementary health approaches in the country. It is also regulated in all 50 states, and chiropractors must complete rigorous educational and licensing requirements.

In Canada, chiropractic has also become a popular healthcare option. The Canadian Chiropractic Association reports that chiropractors are regulated in all provinces and territories and that over four million Canadians visit a chiropractor each year.

In Europe, chiropractic has been slower to gain acceptance, with some countries not fully recognizing it as a healthcare profession. However, in countries like Denmark and Switzerland, chiropractic is a well-established and respected healthcare option. In Denmark, chiropractors are licensed to diagnose and treat musculoskeletal conditions, while in Switzerland, chiropractic is covered by national health insurance.

In Australia, chiropractic is a regulated healthcare profession that is recognized by the government. Chiropractors in Australia must be registered with the Chiropractic Board of Australia and complete continuing education requirements to maintain their registration.

In Asia, chiropractic is becoming more widely recognized, with chiropractors practicing in countries like Japan, South Korea, and Singapore. In Japan, chiropractic is regulated by the government, and chiropractors must complete a four-year program at a recognized chiropractic college. In South Korea, chiropractic has gained popularity among athletes, and chiropractors often work with sports teams to improve performance and prevent injuries. In Singapore, chiropractic is recognized as a complementary therapy and is regulated by the government.

In Africa, chiropractic is still a relatively new healthcare option, but it is gaining popularity. In South Africa, chiropractors are regulated by the Allied Health Professions Council of South Africa and are required to complete a five-year program at an accredited chiropractic college.

In South America, chiropractic is also gaining popularity, with chiropractors practicing in countries like Brazil, Argentina, and Chile. In Brazil, chiropractic is a regulated healthcare profession, and chiropractors must be licensed by the Federal Council of Chiropractic. In Argentina, chiropractic is recognized as a complementary therapy, and chiropractors are regulated by the Ministry of Health.

The global future of chiropractic

Chiropractic is a form of alternative medicine that focuses on the diagnosis, treatment, and prevention of musculoskeletal system disorders, particularly those involving the spine. The practice has been growing in popularity in recent years, and it is becoming increasingly recognized as a viable treatment option for a wide range of conditions. While chiropractic is primarily associated with the United States, it is practiced in various countries around the world, and the field is experiencing significant growth globally.

The history of chiropractic can be traced back to the late 1800s in the United States, where it was developed by Daniel David Palmer. However, it wasn't until the early 1900s that the profession began to gain recognition and acceptance as a legitimate healthcare option. In 1895, Palmer made the first chiropractic adjustment on a patient, which he claimed cured the man's deafness. From that point forward, Palmer and his son, B.J. Palmer, worked to develop and refine the practice of chiropractic.

Today, chiropractic is recognized as a licensed healthcare profession in over 40 countries around the world. In some countries, such as Canada and the United States, chiropractors are considered primary healthcare providers and can diagnose and treat patients without a referral from a medical doctor. In other countries, such as the United Kingdom and Australia, chiropractors are considered complementary or alternative healthcare providers and work in conjunction with medical doctors.

The growth of chiropractic globally can be attributed to a number of factors, including increased public awareness of the benefits of chiropractic, the growing acceptance of alternative and complementary medicine, and the aging population. Many patients seek out chiropractic care for musculoskeletal pain, but the practice is also used for a wide range of other conditions, including headaches, allergies, and digestive problems.

In many countries, chiropractors work in multidisciplinary healthcare teams alongside medical doctors and other healthcare professionals. This collaboration helps to ensure that patients receive the most appropriate and effective treatment for their specific conditions. Additionally, many chiropractors are involved in research and education, contributing to the advancement of the field and the development of new techniques and treatment methods.

The future of chiropractic around the world looks promising. As more research is conducted and the benefits of chiropractic become more widely known, it is likely that more people will seek out chiropractic care as a primary or complementary healthcare option. Furthermore, the increasing focus on holistic and integrated healthcare is expected to drive the demand for chiropractic services.

However, there are also challenges facing the field of chiropractic as it continues to expand globally. One challenge is ensuring that the standards of education and practice are consistent across countries. There are currently no international standards for chiropractic education, and requirements for licensing and practice can vary widely from country to country. Additionally, there is a need for increased communication and collaboration between chiropractors and other healthcare professionals to ensure that patients receive the best possible care.

Chapter Twenty-Four

Patient Stories and Testimonials

Chiropractic is a healthcare profession that focuses on the diagnosis and treatment of musculoskeletal disorders, particularly those affecting the spine. While chiropractic care has gained acceptance as an effective treatment option for a variety of conditions, it is not uncommon for patients to initially seek care with some skepticism. However, many patients have shared their positive experiences with chiropractic care and how it has helped them overcome their health issues.

One common type of testimonial is from patients who have experienced relief from back pain. Back pain is one of the most common reasons that people seek chiropractic care. Patients often report that they have been suffering from chronic back pain for months or even years before seeking chiropractic treatment. In many cases, these patients report that they experience significant improvement in their pain levels after just a few sessions with a chiropractor. They also report being able to engage in activities that they were previously unable to do because of their pain.

Another type of testimonial comes from athletes who have incorporated chiropractic care into their training regimen. Athletes often subject their bodies to intense physical stress and can be at risk for injuries. Many professional athletes have credited chiropractic care with helping them to recover from injuries and improve their performance. Chiropractic care can help athletes maintain proper alignment and joint mobility, which can help prevent injuries from occurring.

Pregnant women also often share their positive experiences with chiropractic care. Pregnancy can put a significant strain on a woman's body, particularly on her back and hips. Chiropractors can use techniques such as the Webster technique to help alleviate pain and discomfort during pregnancy. This technique can also help to optimize the position of the baby for birth.

Patients with chronic headaches and migraines often share stories of how chiropractic care has helped them. Headaches and migraines can be debilitating and have a significant impact on a person's quality of life. Chiropractors can use spinal manipulation and other techniques to help alleviate the pain associated with these conditions.

Patients with conditions such as fibromyalgia and arthritis have also reported positive experiences with chiropractic care. These conditions can be difficult to manage and can cause significant pain and discomfort. Chiropractors can work with patients to develop a treatment plan that includes both chiropractic care and other complementary therapies to help manage their symptoms.

In addition to these specific conditions, patients often report overall improvements in their health and well-being after receiving chiropractic care. Chiropractic care focuses on maintaining proper alignment and mobility in the musculoskeletal system, which can have a positive impact on a person's overall health. Patients often report improved energy levels, better sleep, and an overall sense of well-being after receiving chiropractic care.

While patient stories and testimonials can be a powerful way to communicate the benefits of chiropractic care, it is important to note that individual experiences can vary. Chiropractic care is not a one-size-fits-all treatment and what works for one patient may not work for another. Additionally, it is important for patients to seek care from a licensed and qualified chiropractor who can develop a customized treatment plan based on their specific needs.

Real-life experiences

Chiropractic care has been around for over a century, and over the years, it has helped countless individuals manage and overcome various health conditions. While there are many studies that support the efficacy of chiropractic treatment, personal testimonials from patients can also provide valuable insight into the real-life experiences of individuals who have sought chiropractic care.

One of the most common reasons people seek chiropractic care is to alleviate back and neck pain. Many individuals have found relief from chronic pain through chiropractic adjustments. For example, a patient named Sarah had been struggling with neck and shoulder pain for over a year, which was affecting her work and daily life. She had tried various painkillers and physical therapy, but nothing seemed to help. After receiving chiropractic adjustments, she noticed significant improvement in her pain and range of motion. She was able to return to her normal activities without discomfort.

Another patient, John, suffered from chronic lower back pain for several years. He had undergone surgery, but the pain persisted. He decided to try chiropractic care and noticed a significant improvement in his symptoms after just a few sessions. He continued regular adjustments and was eventually able to stop taking pain medication altogether.

Chiropractic care has also been shown to benefit individuals with other health conditions. For instance, a patient named Alex had been experiencing frequent headaches and migraines for years. She had tried various medications and therapies, but the pain persisted. After a few chiropractic-tic sessions, she noticed a decrease in the frequency and severity of her headaches. Over time, her headaches disappeared altogether.

In addition to physical health conditions, chiropractic care can also benefit individuals with mental health issues. A patient named Lisa had been experiencing anxiety and depression for years, and traditional therapies had not helped her. She decided to try chiropractic care, and over time, she noticed a significant improvement in her symptoms. She felt more relaxed, calmer, and happier overall.

While personal stories like these can be powerful, it is important to note that not all patients will have the same experience with chiropractic care. Each individual's health condition and response to treatment is unique, and results may vary. It is also important to seek care from a licensed and experienced chiropractor to ensure safe and effective treatment.

Success stories and transformations

Chiropractic care has gained a reputation as an effective alternative to traditional medical treatments for a range of conditions, from back pain and headaches to sports injuries and stress-related issues. While there is ongoing debate about the scientific validity of chiropractic, many people around the world have shared their success stories and transformational experiences after seeking care from a chiropractor.

One common theme in these stories is the relief of chronic pain. For many patients, chiropractic adjustments have provided long-term relief from chronic pain conditions like sciatica, herniated discs, and arthritis. This is often attributed to the focus on restoring proper alignment and function to the musculoskeletal system, which can alleviate pressure on nerves and joints that cause pain.

In addition to pain relief, chiropractic care has also been credited with improving overall health and well-being. Patients have reported feeling more energized, experiencing fewer headaches and other ailments, and even sleeping better after receiving regular chiropractic adjustments. This is often attributed to the fact that chiropractors focus on treating the root causes of health problems, rather than simply masking symptoms with medication.

Many athletes have also reported success with chiropractic care. Sports injuries can be particularly debilitating, but chiropractors are trained to address these issues through a combination of spinal adjustments, soft tissue therapy, and exercise rehabilitation. By restoring proper function to the musculoskeletal system, chiropractic can help athletes recover faster and return to their sport with less risk of re-injury.

It's not just athletes who benefit from chiropractic care, however. Many people who lead sedentary lifestyles or work in jobs that require prolonged sitting or standing have found relief from the postural issues that can lead to chronic pain and other health problems. Chiropractors can provide guidance on proper posture and ergonomics, as well as prescribe exercises and stretches to help maintain healthy spinal alignment.

In addition to physical benefits, many patients have also reported positive mental and emotional effects from chiropractic care. By reducing stress and promoting relaxation, chiropractic can help improve mood and reduce symptoms of anxiety and depression. This is often attributed to the mind-body connection that is central to chiropractic philosophy.

While chiropractic care is not a panacea and may not work for everyone, the many success stories and transformations that have been shared by patients around the world suggest that it can be a valuable addition to a comprehensive healthcare plan. By focusing on restoring proper function to the musculoskeletal system, chiropractic can provide relief from chronic pain and other health problems, as well as promote overall health and well-being.

The impact of chiropractic on daily life

Chiropractic is a healthcare profession that focuses on the diagnosis, treatment, and prevention of musculoskeletal disorders, with an emphasis on the spine. While chiropractic has traditionally been associated with treating back and neck pain, it can have a significant impact on daily life beyond just alleviating pain. Below we will explore how chiropractic can affect daily life in various ways.

First and foremost, chiropractic can improve physical function. Many patients seek chiropractic care for pain relief, but chiropractors do more than just alleviate pain symptoms. They also focus on restoring proper alignment and function to the musculoskeletal system, which can lead to improved mobility and range of motion. This can have a significant impact on daily activities, such as being able to bend over to tie one's shoes or reach overhead to grab an object from a shelf.

In addition to physical improvements, chiropractic care can also have a positive impact on mental health. Many patients report feeling more relaxed and less stressed after receiving chiropractic adjustments. This may be due to the fact that chiropractic adjustments can help to relieve tension in the muscles and promote better blood flow throughout the body, which can have a calming effect on the nervous system.

Chiropractic care can also improve sleep quality. Sleep is essential for overall health and well-being, and many patients report improved sleep quality after receiving chiropractic adjustments. This may be due to the fact that chiropractic adjustments can help to relieve tension and pain in the body, making it easier to get comfortable and fall asleep.

Another way that chiropractic can impact daily life is by improving athletic performance. Chiropractic adjustments can help to restore proper alignment and function to the musculoskeletal system, which can lead to improved coordination and balance. This can be especially beneficial for athletes who need to be able to perform at their best and avoid injury.

Chiropractic care can also promote overall wellness and prevent future health problems. Regular chiropractic adjustments can help to keep the musculoskeletal system in proper alignment and function, which can prevent future injuries and health problems. This can have a significant impact on daily life by allowing patients to stay active and healthy, and avoid the need for more invasive treatments or medications.

Furthermore, chiropractic can have a positive impact on relationships. Chronic pain can take a toll on personal relationships, causing stress and strain on marriages and family relationships. By providing relief from pain and improving physical function, chiropractic care can help to reduce stress and tension, and promote better communication and overall well-being.

* 9 7 8 1 7 7 6 9 6 8 3 0 5 *

SD - #0045 - 140926 - C0 - 229/152/11 - PB - 9781776968305 - Matt Lamination